Behind the Scenes of a COVID-19 Test: How It Works

Namita

First Printing, 2024

TABLE OF CONTENTS

CHAPTER 1 01

INTRODUCTION ....

ON THE POST-MODERN SCIENTIFIC CONDITION ....

THE BOOM AND BUST OF SCIENTIFIC FADS ARE AN EXPRESSION OF DESIRE FOR A GRAND NARRATIVE ....

SINGLE-CELL SEQUENCING AND TECHNOLOGY OFFER A ROBUST GRAND NARRATIVE ....

THE ABSENCE OF PANDEMIC PREPAREDNESS EFFECTED A GRAND NARRATIVE ....

NASCENT TRANSCRIPTOMICS IS AN UNTAPPED GOLD MINE OF INFORMATION..........

CHALLENGES IN CIRCADIAN RHYTHMS PRECLUDE THEIR ADOPTION AS A GRAND NARRATIVE ....

TECHNOLOGY DEVELOPMENT OFFERS A CLEAR PATH FOR A PHD ....

CHAPTER 2 15

DEVELOPMENT OF A SALIVA-OPTIMIZED RT-LAMP ASSAY FOR SARS-COV-2 ....

INTRODUCTION ....

METHODS ....

RT-LAMP Reactions ....

Control RNA..........

Saliva inactivation..........

Purification..........

qPCR ....

3D Printing ....

RESULTS ....

Lamp Shade Violet (LSV) and modifications to avoid heterogeneity to avoid saliva pH variation ....

Viral Inactivation at 65°C is effective ....

Testing means of purifying RNA from saliva ....

Optimizing salt concentration ....

Optimizing elution and binding times ....

Optimizing wash buffers ....

StickLAMP ....

Performance analysis of StickLAMP ....

DISCUSSION ....

REFERENCES ....

FIGURES AND FIGURE LEGENDS ....

Figure 1. Two comparisons of Phenol Red against LAMPShade Violet for detection of amplification products in RT-LAMP. ....

Figure 2. Evaluation of inactivation of saliva samples at 65C. ....

Figure 3. Investigating and optimizing saliva for purification. ....

Figure 4. Optimizing the concentrations of salt and PEG for RNA purification from saliva. ....

Figure 5. Optimizing the binding and elution times for magnetic bead-based purification using carboxylated beads with 700mM NaCl and 14% PEG, as measured by SARS-CoV-2 RNA recovery through N1 qPCR from contrived saliva samples. ....

Figure 6. A comparison of three washing conditions for RNA purification from saliva using carboxylated beads with 700mM NaCl and 14% PEG, as measured by SARS-CoV-2 RNA recovery by N1 qPCR from contrived saliva samples. ....

Figure 7. Several features of SalivaBeads purification. ....

Figure 8. Performance evaluation of SalivaBeads and StickLAMP. ....

Figure 9. An overview of StickLAMP and further considerations. ....

CHAPTER 3 45

BUTT-SEQ: A NEW METHOD FOR FACILE PROFILING OF TRANSCRIPTION ....

INTRODUCTION ....

RESULTS ....

Butt-Seq is an efficient 3' Nascent RNA end-labeling technique ....

Butt-Seq results are comparable to those from other established methods ....

Butt-Seq is reproducible down to 10,000 cells ....

KL-1 causes pause sites to recede towards the TSS ....

RNAPII positioning and KL-1 sensitivity correlate with subnucleosomal structures of the -nucleosome ....

Butt-Seq identifies differential pausing dynamics between S2 cells and Drosophila heads

Butt-Seq identifies transcriptional dynamics in key circadian genes ....

Butt-Seq recapitulates circadian transcriptional oscillation details ....

DISCUSSION

METHODS

S2 cell culture and KL-1 treatment

Nascent RNA isolation in S2 cells

Nascent RNA isolation in fly heads

Butt-Seq library prep

Butt-Seq Data Processing

Contaminant analysis

Pro-Seq and 3NT-Seq Data Processing

ChIP-Seq Data Processing and Peak Calling

Butt-Seq Pause Analysis

Pause site analysis

Pausing Index Calculation

Motif analysis

mNase-Seq analysis

H2Av ChIP-Seq analysis.

Data normalization

RNA-Seq analysis

Metagene profiles and gene plots

Data Availability

REFERENCES

FIGURES AND FIGURE LEGENDS ....

Figure 1. Butt-Seq measures transcription and is comparable to other transcription analysis methods. ....

Figure 2. Butt-Seq signal is reproducible down to 10,000 cells. ....

Figure 3. Butt-Seq recapitulates pausing dynamics seen in RNAPII ChIP-Seq upon KL-1 treatment. ....

Figure 4. Pausing as assayed by Butt-Seq is correlated with nucleosomal dynamics. ....

Figure 5. Despite low correlation in gene expression, S2 cells and heads share similar pausing features in co-expressed genes. ....

Figure 6. Differential analysis of Butt-Seq in heads and S2 cells reveals a diverse range of transcriptional programs. ....

Figure 7. Butt-Seq exhibits transcriptional cycling of core circadian genes. ....

Figure 8. Butt-Seq recapitulates known transcriptional features of the Circadian clock......

Supplementary Figure 1. Contaminant measures in different techniques. ....

Supplementary Figure 2. Butt-Seq recapitulates known features of pausing. ....

CHAPTER 4 90

DEVELOPMENT AND APPLICATION OF VIBECHECK IN CIRCADIAN TRANSCRIPTOMICS ....

INTRODUCTION ....

RESULTS ....

Identifying a set of intrinsic cyclers..

Developing VibeCheck Framework and Architecture...

VibeCheck is more resistant to noise than existing approaches ....

VibeCheck uncovers intrinsic cyclers in Drosophila heads...

VibeCheck suggests the majority of cycling genes are transcriptionally driven ....

SP1/BRK is a putative transcription complex regulating periodic expression in glia........

VibeCheck identifies common cycling genes across Clock neurons.................................

VibeCheck identifies unique cycling genes across Clock neuron clusters ....

DISCUSSION ....

METHODS ....

RNA-Seq data processing. ....

Cycling Analysis ....

Intersection simulation ....

Training data for VibeCheck ....

VibeCheck data preprocessing...

Model Architecture ....

Synthetic Data Generation ....

ATAC-Seq Preprocessing..

ATAC-Seq differential peak calling and normalization ....

ATAC-Seq Footprinting ....

Motif Analysis ....

REFERENCES ....

FIGURES AND FIGURE LEGENDS ....

Figure 1. Examinations of cycling dynamics..

Figure 2. Identifying common rhythmic genes between RAIN and JTK_Cycle...............

Figure 3. Benchmarking VibeCheck against JTK_Cycle on simulated data......................

Figure 4. Analysis of circadian dynamics in D. Melanogaster heads using VibeCheck and JTK_Cycle. ....

Figure 5. Comparison of oscillations between mRNA and nascent RNA as measured by Butt-Seq. ....

Figure 6. Integrative analysis of ATAC-Seq and RNA-Seq data implies SP1/BRK as putative regulators of oscillating transcription. ....

Figure 7. Brk/Sp1 may be regulators of circadian transcription in astrocyte-like glia. ......

Figure 8. Identification of common cycling genes between different cell types among Clock neurons. ....

Figure 9. Features of cell-type specific cycling genes in Clock neurons ....

CHAPTER 5 129

DISCUSSIONS AND HYPOTHESES ....

What is pausing for? ....

Chromatin topology subtly mediates gene expression and has a seemingly overlooked relationship with polymerase pausing ....

RNA is involved in enhancer-promoter contacts within TADs ....

Stable enhancer-promoter contacts are only found in organisms with promoter-proximal pausing ....

Pause release depletes enhancer-promoter contacts ....

Circadian involvement of polymerase pausing and enhancer-promoter looping is an open question ....

REFERENCES ....

CHAPTER 1

INTRODUCTION

This introduction was very difficult to write. The thesis before you traverses a patchwork quilt of topics – from testing for COVID-19, to transcriptional pausing, to circadian rhythms. As a result, I felt a traditional introduction to a thesis would inevitably feel aimless and disjointed – not to mention it would be largely redundant with the introductions for each individual chapter. Instead of jumping from subject to subject with no cohesion, I thought to take a different tack.

Despite the scattered trajectory of my PhD, I could sense a unifying theme tying it all together. It intermingles some tangentially related scientific background with philosophical musing, so I thought it might serve well as an introduction, albeit a deeply self-indulgent one.

If you wish to learn the background for the topics covered in this thesis, I direct you to the introduction to each individual chapter (maybe a little bit the last three sections, to contextualize each chapter). If you're happy to engage with an exercise in narcissism (or you are obliged to read this; thank you committee members), please plow forward.

On the Post-Modern scientific condition

Science is hard, and it's getting harder. With each passing year, science has been splintering into increasingly insulated domains – with definitions, language, and even modes of thought growing more intricate and esoteric. We were formally warned of this emerging danger as early as 1992, and a study in 2017 has found that things have only gotten worse with time (Hayes, 1992; Plaven-Sigray et al., 2017). These two studies used lexical difficulty as a metric for these growing schisms, and it as I discuss later, I find it to be a deeply appropriate one.

Though I can only speak towards the biological sciences, I expect this trend can be observed across many disciplines; after all, this ever-narrowing specialization is not unique to science. In his work,

The Postmodern Condition, the philosopher Jean-Francois Lyotard describes the loss of the "grand narrative" – where he describes postmodernity (our current state of being) as an "incredulity towards metanarratives" (Lyotard, 1984). Lyotard believed humanity is historically marked by common telos – narratives governing human ambition that united society under its purpose. To him, postmodernity is defined by the realization of progress for its own sake, and the loss of grand justifications such as "the dialectics of spirit, the hermeneutics of meaning, the emancipation of the rational or working subject, or the creation of wealth". Progress was no longer a means to an end, but an end in of itself – dominated by *petits récits* – little narratives.

Within each little narrative is a state of discourse that Lyotard calls, conjuring Wittgenstein, "language games". Words no longer have any exact meaning – instead, they're defined by communal agreement within each little narrative, with no need for any relationship to definitions agreed upon in other little narratives. I believe anyone who has spent any time in biology should find the "little narrative" to be chillingly resonant.

My personal favorite example is the divergent definition of epigenetics. A molecular biologist evoking epigenetics is probably referring to certain elements that regulate gene expression beyond what's encoded in the DNA – DNA methylation and histone marks, for the most part (Huang, 2022). A systems biologist, on the other hand, is likely to be more faithful to Conrad Waddington's original definition – a heritable response to stimulus that maintains generational patterns of gene expression underlying a phenotype (Waddington, 1956). Systems biologists have since expanded Waddington's original definition to include any element that contributes to a regulatory network defining a cellular phenotype – including transcription factors, histone marks, DNA methylation, and anything else that might chip in (Huang, 2022). As anyone who has worked in epigenetics can attest to, when these two little narratives cross paths, barbs and jabs are thrown over failures to obey the rules of the other's language game.

Though science must legitimize itself, it instead appears to be spiraling into increasingly esoteric and insular domains. The Rosbash lab is a good counterexample – we are an interdisciplinary lab that intermingles molecular biology, biochemistry, and neuroscience to great effect. Indeed, where I find myself diverging from Lyotard is that most scientists do not appear to find the postmodern condition to be a desirable state of being, and many clamor for a "grand narrative" behind whose banner they can march.

I can think of a few broad examples to back up this claim.

The boom and bust of scientific fads are an expression of desire for a grand narrative

The past 20 years or so have seen the rise and fall of what I feel to be a very specific type of scientific fad – ones that claim the discovery of novel biophysical mechanisms that offer tantalizing insights and mechanistic explanations for many outstanding mysteries in biology. Lipid rafts and chromosome topology fall under this definition, I think, having overpromised and (debatably) underdelivered – but I don't know much about the former, and I'm still holding out on hope for the latter (Misteli, 2020; Sezgin et al., 2017). Instead, I'll talk about two others: long non-coding RNAs (lncRNAs) and phase separation.

Awareness of functional lncRNAs has existed since the early 1990s, where Xist – a lncRNA that has withstood the test of time – was first characterized (Brockdorff et al., 1992; Brown et al., 1992). Most would agree, though, that lncRNAs only took off as a field in 2007, when a group reported the function of HOX Antisense Intergenic RNA – HOTAIR (though they may have been inspired by the earlier "discovery" of non-coding RNA trithorax response elements in *Drosophila*) (Rinn et al., 2007; Sanchez-Elsner et al., 2006). HOTAIR was reported as a *trans*-acting non-coding RNA that suppressed transcription across a 40 kilobase locus through interactions with

Polycomb Repressive Complex 2 (PRC2).

While this was interesting in of itself, the story to the greater scientific community was the potential for an entirely new class of functional molecule. This story coincided with the introduction of high-throughput sequencing, which made novel RNA discovery easy and accessible to the masses. Thus, a gold rush began. Within a year or two, functional lncRNAs were being described in every field of biology imaginable (funnily enough, a disproportionate number of them appeared to interact with PRC2) (Fiorenzano et al., 2019; Morris & Mattick, 2014).

However, it wasn't long before cracks started to appear. The effects of HOTAIR deletion in mice were unreproducible, and PRC2 was found to bind RNA promiscuously, seemingly to no notable effect (Amandio et al., 2016; Davidovich et al., 2013). Sober retrospection suggests that the lncRNA boom was largely driven by insufficient biochemical rigor – in other words, a failure to appreciate the limits of one's experimental methods – and overgenerous interpretation of minor or non-existent effects (Mattick et al., 2023). Only after the field cooled did appropriate experimental standards emerge.

We witnessed a very similar phenomenon with the rise of liquid-liquid phase separation (LLPS). Though several examples are robust and have survived the test of time – the nucleolus, for one – in 2011, a study was published that suggested such organelles represented a general mechanism exhibited by all sorts of biomolecules, describing LLPS as a mechanism by which cellular molecules could self-organize into membraneless organelles, similar to the nucleolus (Brangwynne et al., 2011; Hyman et al., 2014). The appeal was enormous – it provided a simple and rational explanation for molecular interactions whose behavior and mechanisms previously defied easy experimental dissection (Banani et al., 2017).

Much as with lncRNAs, LLPS was quick to spread across every imaginable field in biology (Banani et al., 2017; Hyman et al., 2014); however, much like lncRNAs once again, sober perspectives revealed that the biochemical foundations underlying many early discoveries in LLPS were insufficient for proving their biological relevance (Alberti et al., 2019; McSwiggen et al., 2019).

At their heyday, these scientific fads offered a grand narrative in biology. The individual little narratives and internally coded language games across disparate fields would be briefly united under a new grand narrative, where they would strive together to define the new space offered by these new biophysical mechanisms. The conclusion from their success, to me, seems obvious: science is not resistant to a grand narrative. On the contrary, it is desperate for one.

However, I find that the introduction of novel biophysical mechanisms has met with mixed success. The most successful grand narratives are the ones born of rigor. The ones born of rigor, I think, are the ones driven by the introduction of new technology.

Single-cell sequencing and technology offer a robust grand narrative

The meteoric rise of single-cell sequencing is evident to anyone currently working in biology. The trajectory across multiple fields in biology is reminiscent of the scientific fads discussed earlier, and the unifying effect it has had confers upon it a well-earned definition as a grand narrative. It is perhaps the most impactful technology in the Rosbash lab during the tenure of my PhD. Thus far, our group has published two studies using single-cell technologies to characterize small subsets of neurons in Drosophila melanogaster and generated countless insights undergoing further scrutiny (Ma et al., 2023; Ma et al., 2021).

Were one to compare the breadth of insights revealed by these grand narratives, single-cell sequencing can certainly stand toe to toe with lncRNAs and LLPS – yet single-cell sequencing will perhaps withstand the test of time a little bit better. Previous fads were defined by an absence of appropriate experimental standards at the onset of their popularity. This is what distinguishes single-cell technology: it is largely built on the application and rigorous optimization of proven and long-existing technologies.

The first single-cell venture by our lab used a plate-based method, CEL-Seq2, which cleverly integrates linear amplification with T7 polymerase with existing RNA library preparation methods to significantly boost the sensitivity of RNA-sequencing (Hashimshony et al., 2016; Ma et al., 2021). T7 RNA polymerase, of course, has existed as a tool since 1980s, and the molecular principles behind RNA-Seq are of a similar era (Ikeda & Richardson, 1986; Nagalakshmi et al., 2008). The second study used droplet microencapsulation of individual cells on the 10x Genomics platform, which incorporates those principles of RNA-seq with microfluidic encapsulation first described in 2000 (Umbanhowar et al., 2000). One might glibly argue that modern single-cell technology is simply a broader application of a technology first conceived of in 1992, when a group microinjected reverse transcriptase into individual rat neurons (Eberwine et al., 1992).

Perhaps the most heavily employed technology in our lab at the time of this writing is SMART-Seq3, whose history and development exemplifies the philosophy uniting the seemingly disparate topics covered in this thesis. As the "3" suggests, SMART-Seq3 experienced multiple iterative rounds of development to achieve its current level of sensitivity and accuracy (Hagemann-Jensen et al., 2020; Picelli et al., 2014). Within each round of development, the fundamental concept behind the technique remains unchanged; the novelty of SMART-Seq3 over SMART-Seq2 is in part derived from a battery of optimizations involving salt concentrations, reaction additives, and polymerase selection, among others. Though such an endeavor may appear to some to be banal, the improvements they report in sensitivity and reproducibility speak otherwise.

It is through such rigorously developed methods that a robust grand narrative can emerge. The desire to understand life on a single-cell level is one that defines the current era of biology. In my time in science, I have found that many take it for granted that established protocols represent a technique in its highest form – yet in my (short) experience, it has been challenging methods, not biology, that has led to the greatest insights in science. The three chapters of this thesis are united in embrace of developing a deep understanding of their methods and pushing them to their greatest degree.

Michael is particularly fond of a quote by Sydney Brenner: "Progress in science depends on new techniques, new discoveries, and new ideas, probably in that order". The depth of truth borne in this quote is one that was revealed to me throughout my degree; thus, the thesis before you is one borne of that notion – a desire to pursue a grand narrative through the development of technology.

The absence of pandemic preparedness effected a grand narrative

The beginnings of the Covid-19 pandemic presented the world with a grand narrative on an unprecedented scale. For a brief moment before the onset of skepticism and conspiracy, humanity was united in its response to an existential threat.

Science was no exception. Amidst shutdowns and social distancing, investigators around the world were motivated by a desire to help – and for many scientists, there was a clear opportunity for them to apply their expertise.

Although PCR diagnostics was a robust and proven technology, it was immediately clear that the infrastructure to support widespread testing, much less community surveillance, was non-existent. Academia was quick to respond, with dozens of labs leveraging their expertise to help find a solution to expand testing capacity.

Some labs introduced novel molecular strategies for detecting viral RNA, such as CRISPR-mediated approaches (Joung et al., 2020). Others focused on finding diagnostic analytes less invasive and less vulnerable to supply-chain shortages than nasopharyngeal swabs, such as saliva (Vogels et al., 2021). However, the method that was subject to the greatest degree of effort was likely loop-mediated isothermal amplification (LAMP).

LAMP, as the name suggests, amplifies DNA at a constant temperature (Notomi et al., 2000). LAMP uses a polymerase with high strand displacement activity and relies on a strand invasion step with a primer to initiate amplification. Each subsequent amplicon contains a stem-loop structure that offers a single-stranded site for subsequent amplification to prime with greater efficiency. With appropriate primers, LAMP exhibits comparable sensitivity and specificity to PCR, except without requiring the burden of a thermal cycler.

The potential was obvious – thermal cyclers were an expensive and specialized piece of equipment representing a rate limiting step in expanding testing capacity, so scientists all over the world were quick to exploit and optimize the technology for Covid-19 diagnostics.

Within a month of the beginning of the pandemic, a consortium had formed consisting of so-inclined scientists (Moore et al., 2021). In addition to thermal cyclers, members of this consortium tackled other diagnostic bottlenecks, such as shortages of RNA purification kits and FDA approval.

The Covid-19 pandemic offered us the most tangible grand narrative in recent history. In addition to the enormous global effort dedicated towards molecular diagnostics, the sheer volume of research done on SARS-CoV-2 – often from labs without much history in virology – serves as testament to this idea ("COVID research: a year of scientific milestones," 2021). My chapter on this topic reflects our response to the COVID pandemic – to help develop a scalable and inexpensive diagnostic test for COVID-19 and beyond. This experience would also be what enabled me to develop Butt-Seq.

Nascent transcriptomics is an untapped gold mine of information

Bulk transcriptomics is now so widespread it might even be considered trite. When examining novel perturbations or conditions, RNA-Seq often acts as the first line of inquiry – but changes in RNA-Seq can obfuscate a mechanistic understanding of changes in transcript abundance. For example, it is unable to distinguish between transcriptional changes and changes in stability.

Soon after the introduction of RNA-Sequencing technology, the idea to sequence biochemically isolated nascent RNA – RNA undergoing active synthesis – was realized (Nechaev et al., 2010; Rodriguez et al., 2013). This technology exists in two forms – whole transcript sequencing, where the entire breadth of a nascent RNA molecule is sequenced, and 3' end sequencing, where the nascent RNA molecule is sequenced from the base most recently synthesized. The former is largely used for transcriptional quantification, while the latter offers high-resolution regulatory information on transcription, such as pausing. However, neither has seen wide-spread adoption in answering biological questions. Instead, nascent transcriptomics has largely been employed to dissect molecular mechanisms of RNA polymerase dynamics (Churchman & Weissman, 2012; Nojima et al., 2016; Nojima et al., 2015).

This lack of adoption may be partially attributed to a simple lack of interest, but it was also simply not an option – existing methods had such high material demands that it was unfeasible to use them to ask questions in biological tissues (Mayer et al., 2015; Nojima et al., 2015). It is here where an opportunity for a new narrative presents itself – the introduction of technology that would enable the measurement of true transcriptomic responses to stimuli and perturbations. Butt-Seq is my contribution to this topic – to create a facile tool for profiling transcription and nascent RNA.

Challenges in Circadian Rhythms preclude their adoption as a grand narrative

The pervasive influence of circadian rhythms across virtually every mechanism of life has long been known but is deeply underappreciated (Patke et al., 2020; Rijo-Ferreira & Takahashi, 2019). Although the 2017 Nobel Prize indicates that it has taken its place as a grand narrative, circadian rhythm studies are still largely relegated to specific investigation by specialized labs (Nelson et al., 2022).

Part of the reason is obvious: circadian studies are expensive and can dramatically inflate costs and labor. However, even if circadian biology was considered to the extent it deserves, challenges exist within the field that preclude its ability to draw biologically relevant conclusions.

Soon after the introduction of high-throughput sequencing technology, investigators realized that to capture oscillating dynamics genome-wide, the field would have to at least double its sampling frequency – yet for the most part, this didn't happen (Hughes et al., 2017). One of the most popular approaches in circadian biology involves comparing the number of oscillating transcripts between conditions or perturbations – yet with insufficient sampling regimes, the extent of changes in oscillation transcripts tends to be greatly exaggerated due to an overabundance of false negatives cyclers causing an abundance of false positive differential cyclers (Pelikan et al., 2022). A simple "sanity check" such as graphing one's purported oscillating genes may have led to some studies to rethink their conclusions (Abruzzi et al., 2021).

The resistance towards doubling sampling frequency is obvious – it more than doubles the amount of effort – labor and money - involved. Thus, if sampling behavior isn't going to change, then one potential solution is to create a tool adapted for low sampling resoltuions. VibeCheck is my attempt to address this: to create a neural network that can recognize oscillating patterns invisible to algorithms but visible to the human observer.

Technology development offers a clear path for a PhD

A recent study suggests that the rate of progress in science has slowed over time, to which they attribute to the loss of "low-hanging fruit" – a statement echoed by many other scientists in anecdotes and gossip (Marder, 2022; Park et al., 2023). The loss of low-hanging fruit has been accompanied by a rise in complexity and breadth, as author lists and figure counts grow year by year. In days past, it was feasible to earn a PhD through focused and meticulous work – primer walking to clone a gene, for example, could occupy upwards of a year. While many degrees are still earned by relentless effort, projects with such clear and directed vision feel increasingly elusive.

However, this thesis is marked by such relentless effort. A handful of novel ideas established the groundwork, but the bulk of this thesis is defined by painstaking and rigorous optimization, with well-defined steps that offered rapid experimental feedback (the latter point was especially important to keep myself motivated).

In my opinion, technology development is what establishes robust grand narratives in science – but this thesis is not going to establish a new grand narrative, though each chapter represents a small effort to contribute towards one. However, perhaps another contribution this thesis might make is to suggest an option for a meandering PhD candidate. Basic science is not over – there is a vast wealth of knowledge to be discovered. However, I am of the belief that we have hit a critical mass of understanding, where the novelty from leveraging basic science into technology may soon outpace the novelty of discovery. More significantly, however, such application, rather than the discovery of basic science offered me a well-defined path for my PhD, and perhaps I would not be alone in this.

REFERENCES

Abruzzi, K. C., Gobet, C., Naef, F., & Rosbash, M. (2021). Comment on "Circadian rhythms in the absence of the clock gene Bmal1". *Science*, *372*(6539). https://doi.org/10.1126/science.abf0922

Alberti, S., Gladfelter, A., & Mittag, T. (2019). Considerations and Challenges in Studying Liquid-Liquid Phase Separation and Biomolecular Condensates. *Cell*, *176*(3), 419-434. https://doi.org/10.1016/j.cell.2018.12.035

Amandio, A. R., Necsulea, A., Joye, E., Mascrez, B., & Duboule, D. (2016). Hotair Is Dispensible for Mouse Development. *PLoS Genet*, *12*(12), e1006232. https://doi.org/10.1371/journal.pgen.1006232

Banani, S. F., Lee, H. O., Hyman, A. A., & Rosen, M. K. (2017). Biomolecular condensates: organizers of cellular biochemistry. *Nat Rev Mol Cell Biol*, *18*(5), 285-298. https://doi.org/10.1038/nrm.2017.7

Brangwynne, C. P., Mitchison, T. J., & Hyman, A. A. (2011). Active liquid-like behavior of nucleoli determines their size and shape in Xenopus laevis oocytes. *Proc Natl Acad Sci U S A*, *108*(11), 4334-4339. https://doi.org/10.1073/pnas.1017150108

Brockdorff, N., Ashworth, A., Kay, G. F., McCabe, V. M., Norris, D. P., Cooper, P. J., Swift, S., & Rastan, S. (1992). The product of the mouse Xist gene is a 15 kb inactive X-specific transcript containing no conserved ORF and located in the nucleus. *Cell*, *71*(3), 515-526. https://doi.org/10.1016/0092-8674(92)90519-i

Brown, C. J., Hendrich, B. D., Rupert, J. L., Lafreniere, R. G., Xing, Y., Lawrence, J., & Willard, H. F. (1992). The human XIST gene: analysis of a 17 kb inactive X-specific RNA that contains conserved repeats and is highly localized within the nucleus. *Cell*, *71*(3), 527-542. https://doi.org/10.1016/0092-8674(92)90520-m

Churchman, L. S., & Weissman, J. S. (2012). Native elongating transcript sequencing (NET-seq). *Curr Protoc Mol Biol*, *Chapter 4*, Unit 4 14 11-17. https://doi.org/10.1002/0471142727.mb0414s98

COVID research: a year of scientific milestones. (2021). *Nature*. https://doi.org/10.1038/d41586-020-00502-w

Davidovich, C., Zheng, L., Goodrich, K. J., & Cech, T. R. (2013). Promiscuous RNA binding by Polycomb repressive complex 2. *Nat Struct Mol Biol*, *20*(11), 1250-1257. https://doi.org/10.1038/nsmb.2679

Eberwine, J., Yeh, H., Miyashiro, K., Cao, Y., Nair, S., Finnell, R., Zettel, M., & Coleman, P. (1992). Analysis of gene expression in single live neurons. *Proc Natl Acad Sci U S A*, *89*(7), 3010-3014. https://doi.org/10.1073/pnas.89.7.3010

Fiorenzano, A., Pascale, E., Patriarca, E. J., Minchiotti, G., & Fico, A. (2019). LncRNAs and PRC2: Coupled Partners in Embryonic Stem Cells. *Epigenomes*, *3*(3). https://doi.org/10.3390/epigenomes3030014

Hagemann-Jensen, M., Ziegenhain, C., Chen, P., Ramskold, D., Hendriks, G. J., Larsson, A. J. M., Faridani, O. R., & Sandberg, R. (2020). Single-cell RNA counting at allele and isoform resolution using Smart-seq3. *Nat Biotechnol*, *38*(6), 708-714. https://doi.org/10.1038/s41587-020-0497-0

Hashimshony, T., Senderovich, N., Avital, G., Klochendler, A., de Leeuw, Y., Anavy, L., Gennert, D., Li, S., Livak, K. J., Rozenblatt-Rosen, O., Dor, Y., Regev, A., & Yanai, I. (2016). CEL-Seq2: sensitive highly-multiplexed single-cell RNA-Seq. *Genome Biol*, *17*, 77. https://doi.org/10.1186/s13059-016-0938-8

Hayes, D. P. (1992). The growing inaccessibility of science. *Nature*, *356*(6372), 739-740. https://doi.org/10.1038/356739a0

Huang, S. (2022). Towards a unification of the 2 meanings of "epigenetics". *PLoS Biol*, *20*(12), e3001944. https://doi.org/10.1371/journal.pbio.3001944

Hughes, M. E., Abruzzi, K. C., Allada, R., Anafi, R., Arpat, A. B., Asher, G., Baldi, P., de Bekker, C., Bell-Pedersen, D., Blau, J., Brown, S., Ceriani, M. F., Chen, Z., Chiu, J. C., Cox, J., Crowell, A. M., DeBruyne, J. P., Dijk, D. J., DiTacchio, L., . . . Hogenesch, J. B. (2017). Guidelines for Genome-Scale Analysis of Biological Rhythms. *J Biol Rhythms*, *32*(5), 380-393. https://doi.org/10.1177/0748730417728663

Hyman, A. A., Weber, C. A., & Julicher, F. (2014). Liquid-liquid phase separation in biology. *Annu Rev Cell Dev Biol*, *30*, 39-58. https://doi.org/10.1146/annurev-cellbio-100913-013325

Ikeda, R. A., & Richardson, C. C. (1986). Interactions of the RNA polymerase of bacteriophage T7 with its promoter during binding and initiation of transcription. *Proc Natl Acad Sci U S A*, *83*(11), 3614-3618. https://doi.org/10.1073/pnas.83.11.3614

Joung, J., Ladha, A., Saito, M., Kim, N. G., Woolley, A. E., Segel, M., Barretto, R. P. J., Ranu, A., Macrae, R. K., Faure, G., Ioannidi, E. I., Krajeski, R. N., Bruneau, R., Huang, M. W., Yu, X. G., Li, J. Z., Walker, B. D., Hung, D. T., Greninger, A. L., . . . Zhang, F. (2020). Detection of SARS-CoV-2 with SHERLOCK One-Pot Testing. *N Engl J Med*, *383*(15), 1492-1494. https://doi.org/10.1056/NEJMc2026172

Lyotard, J. F. (1984). *The postmodern condition : a report on knowledge / Jean-Francois Lyotard ; translation from the French by Geoff Bennington and Brian Massumi ; foreword by Fredric Jameson*. University of Minnesota Press.

Ma, D., Herndon, N., Le, J. Q., Abruzzi, K. C., Zinn, K., & Rosbash, M. (2023). Neural connectivity molecules best identify the heterogeneous clock and dopaminergic cell types in the Drosophila adult brain. *Sci Adv*, *9*(8), eade8500. https://doi.org/10.1126/sciadv.ade8500

Ma, D., Przybylski, D., Abruzzi, K. C., Schlichting, M., Li, Q., Long, X., & Rosbash, M. (2021). A transcriptomic taxonomy of Drosophila circadian neurons around the clock. *Elife*, *10*. https://doi.org/10.7554/eLife.63056

Marder, E. (2022). Maintaining the joy of discovery. *Elife*, *11*. https://doi.org/10.7554/eLife.80711

Mattick, J. S., Amaral, P. P., Carninci, P., Carpenter, S., Chang, H. Y., Chen, L. L., Chen, R., Dean, C., Dinger, M. E., Fitzgerald, K. A., Gingeras, T. R., Guttman, M., Hirose, T., Huarte, M., Johnson, R., Kanduri, C., Kapranov, P., Lawrence, J. B., Lee, J. T., . . . Wu, M. (2023). Long non-coding RNAs: definitions, functions, challenges and recommendations. *Nat Rev Mol Cell Biol*, *24*(6), 430-447. https://doi.org/10.1038/s41580-022-00566-8

Mayer, A., di Iulio, J., Maleri, S., Eser, U., Vierstra, J., Reynolds, A., Sandstrom, R., Stamatoyannopoulos, J. A., & Churchman, L. S. (2015). Native elongating transcript sequencing reveals human transcriptional activity at nucleotide resolution. *Cell*, *161*(3), 541-554. https://doi.org/10.1016/j.cell.2015.03.010

McSwiggen, D. T., Mir, M., Darzacq, X., & Tjian, R. (2019). Evaluating phase separation in live cells: diagnosis, caveats, and functional consequences. *Genes Dev*, *33*(23-24), 1619-1634. https://doi.org/10.1101/gad.331520.119

Misteli, T. (2020). The Self-Organizing Genome: Principles of Genome Architecture and Function. *Cell*, *183*(1), 28-45. https://doi.org/10.1016/j.cell.2020.09.014

Moore, K. J. M., Cahill, J., Aidelberg, G., Aronoff, R., Bektas, A., Bezdan, D., Butler, D. J., Chittur, S. V., Codyre, M., Federici, F., Tanner, N. A., Tighe, S. W., True, R., Ware, S. B., Wyllie, A. L., Afshin, E. E., Bendesky, A., Chang, C. B., Dela Rosa, R., 2nd, . . . g, L. C. (2021). Loop-Mediated Isothermal Amplification Detection of SARS-CoV-2 and Myriad Other Applications. *J Biomol Tech*, *32*(3), 228-275. https://doi.org/10.7171/jbt.21-3203-017

Morris, K. V., & Mattick, J. S. (2014). The rise of regulatory RNA. *Nat Rev Genet*, *15*(6), 423-437. https://doi.org/10.1038/nrg3722

Nagalakshmi, U., Wang, Z., Waern, K., Shou, C., Raha, D., Gerstein, M., & Snyder, M. (2008). The transcriptional landscape of the yeast genome defined by RNA sequencing. *Science*, *320*(5881), 1344-1349. https://doi.org/10.1126/science.1158441

Nechaev, S., Fargo, D. C., dos Santos, G., Liu, L., Gao, Y., & Adelman, K. (2010). Global analysis of short RNAs reveals widespread promoter-proximal stalling and arrest of Pol II in Drosophila. *Science*, *327*(5963), 335-338. https://doi.org/10.1126/science.1181421

Nelson, R. J., Bumgarner, J. R., Liu, J. A., Love, J. A., Melendez-Fernandez, O. H., Becker-Krail, D. D., Walker, W. H., 2nd, Walton, J. C., DeVries, A. C., & Prendergast, B. J. (2022). Time of day as a critical variable in biology. *BMC Biol*, *20*(1), 142. https://doi.org/10.1186/s12915-022-01333-z

Nojima, T., Gomes, T., Carmo-Fonseca, M., & Proudfoot, N. J. (2016). Mammalian NET-seq analysis defines nascent RNA profiles and associated RNA processing genome-wide. *Nat Protoc*, *11*(3), 413-428. https://doi.org/10.1038/nprot.2016.012

Nojima, T., Gomes, T., Grosso, A. R. F., Kimura, H., Dye, M. J., Dhir, S., Carmo-Fonseca, M., & Proudfoot, N. J. (2015). Mammalian NET-Seq Reveals Genome-wide Nascent Transcription Coupled to RNA Processing. *Cell*, *161*(3), 526-540. https://doi.org/10.1016/j.cell.2015.03.027

Notomi, T., Okayama, H., Masubuchi, H., Yonekawa, T., Watanabe, K., Amino, N., & Hase, T. (2000). Loop-mediated isothermal amplification of DNA. *Nucleic Acids Res*, *28*(12), E63. https://doi.org/10.1093/nar/28.12.e63

Park, M., Leahey, E., & Funk, R. J. (2023). Papers and patents are becoming less disruptive over time. *Nature*, *613*(7942), 138-144. https://doi.org/10.1038/s41586-022-05543-x

Patke, A., Young, M. W., & Axelrod, S. (2020). Molecular mechanisms and physiological importance of circadian rhythms. *Nat Rev Mol Cell Biol*, *21*(2), 67-84. https://doi.org/10.1038/s41580-019-0179-2

Pelikan, A., Herzel, H., Kramer, A., & Ananthasubramaniam, B. (2022). Venn diagram analysis overestimates the extent of circadian rhythm reprogramming. *FEBS J*, *289*(21), 6605-6621. https://doi.org/10.1111/febs.16095

Picelli, S., Faridani, O. R., Bjorklund, A. K., Winberg, G., Sagasser, S., & Sandberg, R. (2014). Full-length RNA-seq from single cells using Smart-seq2. *Nat Protoc*, *9*(1), 171-181. https://doi.org/10.1038/nprot.2014.006

Plaven-Sigray, P., Matheson, G. J., Schiffler, B. C., & Thompson, W. H. (2017). The readability of scientific texts is decreasing over time. *Elife*, *6*. https://doi.org/10.7554/eLife.27725

Rijo-Ferreira, F., & Takahashi, J. S. (2019). Genomics of circadian rhythms in health and disease. *Genome Med*, *11*(1), 82. https://doi.org/10.1186/s13073-019-0704-0

Rinn, J. L., Kertesz, M., Wang, J. K., Squazzo, S. L., Xu, X., Brugmann, S. A., Goodnough, L. H., Helms, J. A., Farnham, P. J., Segal, E., & Chang, H. Y. (2007). Functional demarcation of active and silent chromatin domains in human HOX loci by noncoding RNAs. *Cell*, *129*(7), 1311-1323. https://doi.org/10.1016/j.cell.2007.05.022

Rodriguez, J., Tang, C. H., Khodor, Y. L., Vodala, S., Menet, J. S., & Rosbash, M. (2013). Nascent-Seq analysis of Drosophila cycling gene expression. *Proc Natl Acad Sci U S A*, *110*(4), E275-284. https://doi.org/10.1073/pnas.1219969110

Sanchez-Elsner, T., Gou, D., Kremmer, E., & Sauer, F. (2006). Noncoding RNAs of trithorax response elements recruit Drosophila Ash1 to Ultrabithorax. *Science*, *311*(5764), 1118-1123. https://doi.org/10.1126/science.1117705

Sezgin, E., Levental, I., Mayor, S., & Eggeling, C. (2017). The mystery of membrane organization: composition, regulation and roles of lipid rafts. *Nat Rev Mol Cell Biol*, *18*(6), 361-374. https://doi.org/10.1038/nrm.2017.16

Umbanhowar, P. B., Prasad, V., & Weitz, D. A. (2000). Monodisperse Emulsion Generation via Drop Break Off in a Coflowing Stream. *Langmuir*, *16*(2), 347-351. https://doi.org/10.1021/la990101e

Vogels, C. B. F., Watkins, A. E., Harden, C. A., Brackney, D. E., Shafer, J., Wang, J., Caraballo, C., Kalinich, C. C., Ott, I. M., Fauver, J. R., Kudo, E., Lu, P., Venkataraman, A., Tokuyama, M., Moore, A. J., Muenker, M. C., Casanovas-Massana, A., Fournier, J., Bermejo, S., . . . Grubaugh, N. D. (2021). SalivaDirect: A simplified and flexible platform to enhance SARS-CoV-2 testing capacity. *Med*, *2*(3), 263-280 e266. https://doi.org/10.1016/j.medj.2020.12.010

Waddington, C. H. (1956). Genetic assimilation of the bithorax phenotype. *Evolution*, *10*(Mar. 1956), 1-13. https://doi.org/doi.org/10.2307/2406091

CHAPTER 2

Development of a saliva-optimized RT-LAMP assay for SARS-CoV-2

Albert D Yu[1], Kristina Galatsis[1], Jian Zheng[2], Jasmine Quynh Le[1], Dingbang Ma[1], Stanley Perlman[2], Michael Rosbash[1]

[1]Howard Hughes Medical Institute and Department of Biology Brandeis University, Waltham, MA 02454, USA

[2]Department of Microbiology and Immunology, University of Iowa, Iowa City, Iowa, USA

Funding and disclosures: Research was funded by Howard Hughes Medical Institute.

Statement for use of human samples: Research using human saliva was approved by the IRB at Brandeis University.

This work has been published at Journal of Biomolecular Techniques.

J Biomol Tech. 2021 Sep;32(3):102-113. doi: 10.7171/jbt.21-3203-005. PMID: 35027868; PMCID: PMC8730519.

INTRODUCTION

The severe acute respiratory syndrome coronavirus 2 (SARS-CoV-2) pandemic has highlighted many shortcomings in our national response and has driven an enormous increase in our need for in vitro diagnostics. A diagnostic test for SARS-CoV-2 using quantitative real-time polymerase chain reaction (qPCR) technology and nasopharyngeal swabs was developed within weeks of identifying the virus but is suboptimal for serving all diagnostic needs of this global pandemic.

This technology has struggled with turnaround time, supply chain shortages, and cost in the effort to increase the amount of testing worldwide.1 Many entities, commercial and academic alike, have risen to the challenge of adapting and developing molecular technologies to address these shortcomings. Among the myriad efforts that subsequently emerged, reverse transcription loop-mediated isothermal amplification (RT-LAMP) technology may prove to be a viable if not preferable alternative to qPCR technology in addressing at least some of the diagnostic needs of a global pandemic.

LAMP is a nucleic acid detection technology that operates like PCR on the principle of nucleic acid amplification.2 Unlike PCR however, LAMP is an isothermal technology and therefore obviates the need for thermal cyclers that would otherwise gate diagnostics behind equipment that costs several thousand dollars. Briefly, LAMP requires at least four (and up to six) different primers: two that contain a self-complementary region that generates a perpetually single-stranded loop structure as well as two that target the region within the single-stranded loop structure. A strand invasion event with the two self-complementing primers initiates production of the initial product containing open loops at either end; exponential amplification can then occur using the loop-targeting primers and a polymerase with strand-displacement ability. In short, LAMP can generate a detectable amount of DNA in a comparable amount of time to PCR but at a single reaction temperature. The DNA can be detected through several different means, including turbidity or through fluorescence with the inclusion of a fluorescent dye. However, a result interpretable to the naked eye would be optimal for a test to enjoy widespread use.3,4 Earlier efforts have explored the use of colorimetric detection of amplification products using a pH dye, phenol red, or a magnesium indicator, hydroxynaphthol blue (HNB).5–9 With phenol red, the color will change from red to yellow as more DNA acidifies the reaction. With HNB, the color will change from light blue to dark blue in the presence of magnesium which is a byproduct of amplification. These color changes are adequate but suffer from limited visible contrast and can often exhibit ambiguous color changes. Our work here uses the novel pH dye LAMPShade Violet (LSV) as an alternative to phenol red in RT-LAMP.10 LSV has greater visual contrast between high and low pH and a stronger inflection point, both easing interpretation and reducing the number of ambiguous events.

Saliva is growing increasingly popular as an alternative respiratory specimen to nasopharyngeal swabs for the detection of SARS-CoV-2. Saliva is much easier to collect, and some report that it is a comparable, even superior specimen for SARS-CoV-2 diagnostics.11 Previous efforts have identified saliva as compatible with RT-LAMP even in the absence of RNA purification. It was replaced by an inactivation step that normalizes the pH, releases RNA, and inactivates RNases.5 However, saliva is very heterogenous between individuals, which confounds a one-size-fits-all inactivation strategy. We therefore optimized an inactivation protocol with improved success across heterogenous saliva samples when combined with LAMPShade Violet. We suggest that this direct method is suitable for small-scale testing environments where it is easy to resample.

Despite this improvement, many saliva samples were still incompatible with direct input into a colorimetric RT-LAMP reaction. This is prohibitive at scale, where samples cannot be individually resampled or modified for compatibility. We therefore developed and introduced a magnetic bead-based rapid RNA-purification procedure for saliva, which we term "SalivaBeads." It features a saliva-optimized bead binding solution and uses a magnetic stick (MS) to isolate RNA-bound magnetic beads, which not only improves processing time and scalability but also resolves issues surrounding saliva compatibility with colorimetric RT-LAMP. The SalivaBeads procedure also takes less than ten minutes and substantially improves sensitivity over direct input.

This paper therefore describes our efforts to develop and optimize this low-cost, scalable, and sensitive saliva RT-LAMP protocol, which also minimizes reliance on specialized equipment. The MS is an inexpensive and dramatically more scalable alternative for RNA purification from saliva compared to magnetic racks and multichannel pipettes. We also improved several previous efforts with enhanced visual fidelity, sample compatibility, and sensitivity at minimal additional cost. Altogether, our protocol exhibits a limit of detection of 3.7 copies/μl in a 200μl saliva sample, costs less than $5 per sample without pooling or accounting for labor and takes approximately 1 hour to conduct from beginning to end.

METHODS

RT-LAMP Reactions

Phenol Red experiments were conducted using WarmStart Colorimetric LAMP 2x Master Mix (New England Biolabs (NEB), M1800L) in 25μl reactions with 5μl of inactivated saliva. Lampshade violet experiments were conducted using a buffer consisting of 5mM Tris ph8.5, 8mM MgSO4, 30mM KCl, 0.1% Tween-20, 10mM dNTPs, 12.5mM KOH, 10mM LampShade Violet10(Luke Lavis, Janelia Research Labs), 0.5μl Warmstart RTx Reverse Transcriptase (NEB M0380L), Bst 2.0 WarmStart DNA Polymerase (NEB M0538L) in 25μl reactions with 5μl of inactivated saliva. For magnetic stick experiments, SARS-CoV-2 reactions were conducted in 25μl reactions, while Actin reactions were conducted in 20μl. All reactions were heated to 65°C for 45 minutes and cooled to at least room temperature prior to examination. Table 1 describes primer sequences and concentrations used to produce a 5x primer solution. Primer sequences are derived from previous work4,5.

Reactions were imaged on an Epson V850 Scanner.

Table 1 Primers used in study.

Concentration	Component	Sequence
1µM	E1-F3	TGAGTACGAACTTATGTACTCAT
1µM	E1-B3	TTCAGATTTTTAACACGAGAGT
8µM	E1-FIP	ACCACGAAAGCAAGAAAAAGAAGTTCGTTTCGGAAGAGACAG
8µM	E1-BIP	TTGCTAGTTACACTAGCCATCCTTAGGTTTTACAAGACTCACGT
2µM	E1-LB	GCGCTTCGATTGTGTGCGT
2µM	E1-LF	CGCTATTAACTATTAACG
1µM	Orf1a-HMS-F3	CGGTGGACAAATTGTCAC
1µM	Orf1a-HMS-B3	CTTCTCTGGATTTAACACACTT
8µM	Orf1a-HMS-LF	TTACAAGCTTAAAGAATGTCTGAACACT
8µM	Orf1a-HMS-LB	TTGAATTTAGGTGAAACATTTGTCACG
2µM	Orf1a-HMSe-FIP	TCAGCACACAAAGCCAAAAATTTATTTTCTGTGCAAAGGAAATTAAGGAG
2µM	Orf1a-HMSe-BIP	TATTGGTGGAGCTAAACTTAAAGCCTTTTCTGTACAATCCCTTTGAGTG

Control RNA

Contrived samples were created using either heat-inactivated SARS-CoV-2 RNA from BEI (NR-52286), or inactivated SARS-CoV-2 viral particles from Zeptometrix (CAT# NATSARS(COV2)-ST). To optimize and evaluate magnetic-bead purification procedures, RNA from The Biodefense and Emerging Infections Research Resources Repository (BEI Resources) was diluted in 1ng/µl Drosophila RNA to 1000 copies/µl and spiked in to inactivated saliva at the stated concentration. In order to evaluate the full-process performance of the protocol, limit of detection experiments and experiments intended to evaluate RNA release fom viral particles were conducted using Zeptometrix SARS-CoV-2 particles added into raw saliva at the stated concentrations. In the proceeding methods, the control used will be specified.

Saliva inactivation

10x inactivation was prepared with 62.5mM tris(2-carboxyethyl)phosphine (TCEP)(Goldbio TCEP1), 10mM EDTA (ThermoFisher Scientific 10977015), and 130mM NaOH. 10x inactivation reagent was added to a final concentration of 1x to raw saliva and inverted 10 times, or vortexed for 5 seconds at maximum speed. Saliva samples were then heated to 95°C for 5 minutes and allowed to cool at room temperature for 3 minutes prior to downstream processing. When testing 65°C inactivation, we inactivated for 15 minutes at 65°C and let samples cool to room temperature for 3 minutes prior to downstream processing. During optimization experiments, TCEP concentrations used are as described in Fig. 3B and results. During Proteinase K testing, the indicated amount of Proteinase K (NEB P8107S) was added to saliva and heated at 65°C for 5 minutes and inactivated at 95°C for 10 minutes. Virus titers in untreated or treated samples were then determined using Vero E6 cells (grown in 10% Fetal Bovine Serum(FBS)-Dulbeccos Modified Eagle Medium(DMEM)). For plaque assays, cells were fixed with 10% formaldehyde 3 days after infection and stained with crystal violet.

Purification

Commercial Ampure XP beads (Beckman-Coulter Life Sciences A63881) were used according to protocol at 2x volumes and eluted in 30μl Milli-Q H2O.

Unmodified homemade magnetic bead buffer was prepared using 100mM NaCl (Sigma-Aldrich S9888), 20% PEG-8000 w/v (Sigma-Aldrich 1546605), 10mM Tris-HCl, pH 8, 1mM EDTA (ThermoFisher Scientific 10977015, and Milli-Q H2O to 50ml. 1000μl Sera-mag Speedbeads (FisherScientific 09-981-123) were washed twice in 1ml 10mM Tris ph 8, 1mM EDTA, and added to bead buffer. The final SalivaBeads recipe uses the same materials as listed above, but with 700mM NaCl, 14% PEG-8000 w/v, 10mM Tris-HCl, pH8, 1mM EDTA, 200μl Sera-mag Speedbeads, and Milli-Q H2O to 50ml. Commercial Ampure XP beads and unmodified homemade magnetic bead buffer was used according to commercial Ampure XP protocols.

For Salivabeads, two volumes of SalivaBeads were added to inactivated saliva samples and inverted 5 times. Bead+saliva mix was incubated at room temperature for 3 minutes. A magnetic stick with tip was added to bead+saliva mix for two minutes, with agitation at one minute and before removing. Magnetic stick with bound beads were dipped in 100μl Milli-Q H2O prepared in a PCR strip tube up and down 5 times, then left to incubate for 20-25 seconds. The magnetic stick was then removed from the water and placed in SARS-CoV-2 reaction mix for 60 seconds. After 60 seconds, the magnetic stick was removed from the SARS-CoV-2 reaction mix and placed in Actin reaction mix for 30 seconds, then removed and the tip was discarded.

For purifying RNA from wash steps, ethanol was added to each sample to a final concentration of 75% and a final volume of 200μl. Sodium acetate (Invitrogen AM9740) was added to a final concentration of 0.3M. Samples were left to precipitate overnight at -20°C. The next day, samples were spun down for 30 minutes at 18000xg relative centrifugal force (RCF). Samples were washed once in 80% ethanol and eluted into 20μl of Milli-Q H2O, 5μl of which was subsequently used in qPCR reactions.

qPCR

qPCR was done using Luna Universal Probe One-Step RT-qPCR Kit (NEB E3006L) and the CDC N1 primer (IDT 10006713). Reactions and cycling conditions were prepared according to manufacturer's protocol.

3D Printing

Magnetic Sticks and Tips were printed using Siraya Tech Blu (Siraya Tech) on an Epax X10 UV LCD 3D Printer with 8.9 inch 4K mono LCD (Epax) using the following settings: 0.05mm Layer Height, 8 Bottom Layers, 3.2s Exposure Time, 12.4s Bottom Exposure Time, 7mm Lift, 35mm/min Lift Speed, 125mm/min Retract Speed. Magnets used were 2.54mm Diameter, 0.600" Length N50 magnets (SuperMagnetMan, Cyl0072-20).

RESULTS

We present two different SARS-CoV-2 protocols. The first, named "the direct assay" is conducted on inactivated, unpurified saliva; it is suitable for low throughput testing in low resource environments. However, high frequency or large population testing is likely to prove problematic. This is in part due to the pH variation exhibited by different sources of saliva. In order to address this issue, we developed a second version, "the purified assay", which adds a novel and rapid purification step. It normalizes saliva pH from different sources while improving sensitivity.

Both protocols begin identically: the crude saliva samples are inactivated by addition of TCEP, EDTA, and NaOH solution. The samples are then heated to 95°C for 5 minutes and allowed to cool at room temperature for at least 3 minutes. In the direct assay, 5μl of inactivated saliva is then added to two RT-LAMP reactions, one targeting SARS-CoV-2 and the other actin. In the purified assay, 2 volumes of SalivaBeads – described below - are added for 5 minutes before being removed by a magnetic stick. The stick-bound beads are washed in water for 30 seconds and then eluted twice sequentially, first directly into a SARS-CoV-2 RT-LAMP reaction and then into an actin RT-LAMP reaction. In both assays, RT-LAMP reactions are incubated at 65°C for 45 minutes.

Both assays rely on the color difference caused by successful DNA amplification. A positive test is indicated by both reactions turning clear, a negative test is indicated by the actin reaction turning clear and the SARS-CoV-2 reaction remaining purple, and an inconclusive/unsuccessful test is indicated by the Actin reaction remaining purple. Comparing the color changes in the two reactions is critical in the direct assay, where baseline color may be affected by the pH of the input saliva sample. However, a careful comparison is less important is the purified assay, where all samples exhibit comparable baseline pH values following purification. What follows describes our efforts in developing and optimizing the parameters of our protocol.

Lamp Shade Violet (LSV) and modifications to avoid heterogeneity to avoid saliva pH variation

In our initial tests, we used a previously described 100x inactivation reagent consisting of 2.5M TCEP, 100mM EDTA, and 1.2M NaOH.5 The NaOH concentration is critical, as the colorimetric readout varies with pH. As in this publication,5 we initially used the colorimetric RT-LAMP reagent provided by NEB, which use Phenol Red as a pH sensor. Phenol Red changes from red to yellow upon acidification by successful amplification.

Although 1.2M NaOH was sufficient in most cases, many samples were still too acidic and caused the reaction to turn prematurely positive, meaning even prior to incubation. To address this problem, we took two approaches which were evaluated on four different samples from four individuals (Fig. 1A). First, we increased the NaOH concentration to 1.4M and 1.6M and observed the color changes pre- and post- incubation. Second, we used a different pH-sensitive dye – LAMPShade Violet (LSV).10 It changes from purple to clear upon successful amplification. Because LSV has sharper contrast and fewer intermediate color changes than Phenol Red, we hypothesized that LSV may help with the interpretation of samples from saliva with outlier pH values.

1.4M NaOH was the best concentration to accommodate samples across different pH values. Although a color difference was observed between positive and negatives samples, more alkaline samples were still ambiguous with Phenol Red. LAMPShade Violet in contrast was superior in distinguishing positive and negative samples.

To compare our in-house RT-LAMP reaction to NEB-supplied reagents, we used them both to detect 20 copies of SARS-CoV-2 RNA, which is near the threshold for success (Fig. 1B). They were qualitatively similar: our in-house version was positive 5 out of 8 times, whereas the commercial was positive 4 out of 8 times. Yet we prefer LSV because of its superior contrast and performance with samples of heterogenous pH values.

Viral Inactivation at 65°C is effective

The current protocol involves virus inactivation at 95°C followed by a 65°C RT-LAMP incubation. To simplify the protocol and further reduce equipment demands, we assayed virus inactivation at 65°C or even at room temperature (RT) with or without inactivation reagent.

Whereas 5 min at RT was insufficient to eliminate biological activity even with the addition of inactivation reagent, 5 min at 65°C with or without reagent addition reduced activity to undetectable, i.e., by at least 5-6 log units (Fig. 2A).

We also compared SARS-CoV-2 RNA yield from a 65°C vs a 95°C incubation. To create specimens that most closely resembled clinical samples, we contrived saliva samples using inactivated but intact SARS-CoV-2 virions from Zeptometrix (Fig. 2B). A 65°C degree inactivation for 15 minutes led to a significant 1-cycle, approximately 2-fold loss in RNA yield compared to a 95°C inactivation for 5 min ($t(4)=3.274$, $p=0.0307$). This modest decrease suggests that 65°C inactivation is an acceptable alternative in environments that can only afford minimal equipment or are otherwise averse to near-boiling temperatures. However, the improvement in yield at 95°C suggests that it is preferred in environments that can accommodate this temperature. Further efforts described below use this inactivation temperature.

Testing means of purifying RNA from saliva

To further improve sensitivity and sample compatibility, we sought to develop a rapid RNA purification protocol optimized for saliva. We first measured RNA recovery using fluorimetry with a Qubit device and compared various bead-based methods with Trizol purification (Fig. 3A). They included: 2 volumes of Ampure Beads XP, 2 volumes of magnetic silica beads in an NaCl/PEG-8000 solution, 2 volumes of magnetic carboxylated beads in an NaCl/PEG-8000 solution, glass milk in a NaCl/PEG-8000 solution as well as glass milk in a Sodium Iodide (NaI) solution as previously described.5,12 Ampure XP beads as well as the NaCl/PEG-8000 based bead mixes were comparable to Trizol (Fig. 3A). Due to lower cost and the advantage of being suitable for scale and automation, we decided to use the NaCl/PEG-8000 based bead mix with carboxylated beads for further optimization of RNA purification from saliva.

Because current inactivation procedures were developed for direct input of saliva into an RT-LAMP reaction, we further optimized inactivation for input into bead-based RNA purification. Different concentrations of TCEP as well as Proteinase K were assayed, the later with a 5 min 65°C incubation followed by a 5 min 95°C incubation (Fig. 3C).

Although Proteinase K was effective in increasing RNA yield compared to the initial condition of 2.5mM TCEP, 6.25mM TCEP was even better and used below.

Optimizing salt concentration

To optimize the NaCl/Peg-8000 bead mix, we examined the effects of salt type, salt concentration, and PEG-8000 concentration on RNA yield from saliva. For reference, the original purification recipe calls for 1M NaCl, and 18% PEG-8000.12 Different concentrations of NaCl and different concentrations of Sodium Acetate (NaOAc) were assayed; the latter is also commonly used in nucleic acid precipitation. Different concentrations of Guanidine Hydrochloride (GuHCl) – another reagent commonly used in nucleic acid purification – were also assessed (Fig. 4A). Although all salts at all concentrations tested could purify RNA, NaCl at a reduced concentration of 0.7M produced a significant higher yield compared to the original recipe at 1M (P<1x10-4, One-Way ANOVA, Tukey's Honest Significance Difference (HSD)) and compared to the other salts.

In other tests, the addition of PEG-8000 to RT-LAMP increased the false positive rate (data not shown). Although we did not see a similar change with the purified assay, it is possible that a modestly increased rate becomes relevant with large scale testing. We therefore decided to reduce the concentration of PEG-8000 until it affected yield. We found no significant difference between 18% PEG-8000 and 12% PEG-8000 (Fig. 4B). Because visual examination of the data suggested a slight loss of sensitivity between 14% and 12% (data not shown), we adjusted the buffer to 14% PEG-8000. Our final adjusted recipe therefore uses 0.7M NaCl and 14% PEG- 8000.

Optimizing elution and binding times

In our purification protocol, the bead mix is left to bind RNA for a certain amount of time before being removed by a magnet, henceforth referred to as binding time. At the end of the protocol, the beads are left to release RNA in the reaction mix for a certain amount of time, henceforth referred to as elution time. Our earlier development procedures used a 5 minute binding time and a 1 minute elution time. To minimize the test processing time, we determined the minimal binding and elution times without sacrificing sensitivity. We first tested a 1 minute, 5 minute, and 15 minute binding time with a 1 minute elution. We observed a significant difference between 1 minute and a 5 minute binding time ($p < 0.01$, One-Way ANOVA, Tukey's HSD) but no significant difference between 5 minutes and 15 minutes (Fig. 5A). We therefore chose a 5 minute binding time. We then compared 10 second, 1 minute, and 5 minute elution time (Fig. 5B). We found no significant differences and so chose an elution time of 30 seconds for improved operational consistency.

Optimizing wash buffers

The majority of bead-based RNA purification protocols feature a 70-80% ethanol (EtOH) wash to remove non-specifically bound contaminants without removing nucleic acids. Because ethanol is incompatible with many downstream enzymatic reactions, protocols involving an ethanol wash typically require a long drying step to remove all traces of ethanol. To eliminate this drying step, we compared this standard 80% ethanol wash to Water and to 130mM NaCl, which was used in a cellulose dipstick-based purification assay.13 We therefore washed the beads for 30 seconds in 200μl of the indicated wash buffers and then eluted in 50μl of Deionized H2O for 30 seconds.

We then ethanol precipitated the RNA under standard conditions (see methods) and assayed recovery by qPCR.

There was no significant difference between RNA levels in the 80% EtOH and in the Water wash fractions (Fig. 6A). However, 130mM NaCl washed off significantly more RNA ($p<1x10-4$, One-Way ANOVA, Tukey's HSD). In the eluate, there was no significant difference between RNA recovered from the 130mM NaCl-washed beads and the 80% EtoH- washed beads, but the H2O-washed beads exhibited a significant 1-cycle improvement ($p<1x10- 3$, One-way ANOVA, Tukey's HSD) (Fig. 6B). We therefore decided that water was the most suitable wash reagent for quick purification, also because water is compatible with the RT- LAMP reaction and requires no drying step following washing.

These changes and optimizations and our bead mix are henceforth referred to as "SalivaBeads".

StickLAMP

Most nucleic acid isolation procedures that use magnetic beads also employ an elution step, which releases the purified RNA into an intermediate buffer such as water or Tris prior to addition to a reaction. We sought to simplify this strategy by eluting RNA from SalivaBeads directly into the RT-LAMP mix. However, the sensitivity was poor compared to the direct assay. Both assays were able to routinely detect 100 copies/μl of SARS-CoV-2 RNA, but only the direct assay was able to detect 25 copies/μl. (Fig. 7A).

To address whether this was due to a poor RNA yield from SalivaBeads, we compared this yield to that from Ampure XP beads. This was done from saliva as well as from purified RNA in water

(Fig. 7B). SalivaBeads had superior yield to Ampure XP beads from saliva but inferior from water. Moreover, the SalivaBeads yield from saliva was comparable to the Ampure XP yield from water. This indicates that the reduced sensitivity is not due to poor yield but rather from some sort of contaminant carryover or other incompatibility.

Indeed, we noticed that considerable debris clung to the SalivaBeads that persisted through the wash step and contaminated the RT-LAMP mix (Fig. 7C, left). We therefore developed a magnetic stick that would remove the beads prior to downstream processing (Fig. 7D). Importantly, the stick appeared to be selective for removing the beads without most of the saliva debris (Fig. 7C, right). Consistent with this observation, magnetic stick purification could faithfully detect 10 copies/µl, whereas magnetic rack purification could not (Fig. 7E).

Performance analysis of StickLAMP

To evaluate the performance of StickLAMP purification, we determined the copy number at which 95% of reactions score positive, henceforth referred to as the limit of detection (LOD). Our LOD was at least 3.7 copies per microliter, i.e., 19 of 20 contrived samples with 3.7 copies of SARS-CoV-2/µl in 200ul saliva scored positive (Fig. 8A).

To ensure that this LOD is similar across a wide variety of saliva types, we collected saliva from 16 different individuals and created two contrived samples per individual with 3.7 copies/µl of SARS-CoV-2 (Fig. 8B). For 15/16 individuals, both samples were positive. For the 16th individual, only one sample was positive, but both samples were positive upon retesting. The 3.7 copy/µl LOD is therefore robust across different individuals.

DISCUSSION

We present two protocols for the detection of SARS-CoV-2 RNA from saliva, which feature several innovations. First, LAMPShade Violet (LSV) is an attractive alternative to Phenol Red for the colorimetric detection of SARS-CoV-2 RNA in saliva; LSV improves visual fidelity without sacrificing sensitivity. Second, 65° is completely successful at viral inactivation in saliva. Compared to the more standard 95°C, 65°C enhances safety, reduces testing time and equipment demands with only somewhat reduced detection sensitivity. Third, we present a rapid purification protocol. It adds less than ten minutes to the processing time, costs less than 20 cents per sample, and is optimized for saliva. The purification improves sensitivity over tenfold and normalizes sample pH for downstream colorimetric detection.

Purification uses a magnetic stick (MS) as an integral tool for rapid nucleic acid purification. Saliva contains substantial and variable levels of debris. It sticks to nucleic acid binding media like beads and inhibits the LAMP colorimetric assay. One previous effort also focused on this assay circumvented the debris issue with centrifugation5. However, this solution is undesirable for scaled testing as centrifuges are difficult to introduce into an automated workflow. They are also expensive and are contrary to the goal of minimizing equipment requirements. The MS selectively binds magnetic beads over saliva debris and therefore substitutes for centrifugation. MS also has several advantages over the other traditional method of bead separation, magnetic rack purification.

First, MS has superior scaling potential. Multichannel pipettes are typically used in magnetic rack purification to improve throughput and sample processing time in both manual and automated workflows. Importantly however, the number of channels is constrained by mechanical considerations in multichannel pipettes, whereas the MS simplicity enables the number of simultaneous "channels" to scale well beyond traditional limitations. Indeed, we developed 4-channel, 8-channel, and a 24-channel versions for the purpose of large- scale multiplex purification reactions, as well as a custom rack designed for a 24-channel MS to elute directly into a 96 or 384-well plate (Fig. 9B and 9C). Second, this superior scaling potential also reduces the additional processing time required by more samples. The addition of every 8 samples increases the required processing time with an 8-channel multipipette, but a 24-channel MS increases processing time only beyond 24 samples. The processing time is further reduced because 2-3 pipetting steps are replaced with a single dipping step. Third, the cost of a MS is dramatically less than a multichannel pipette. A 24- channel magnetic stick costs less than \$5.00 to produce, and each tip is less than \$0.05, about \$6.00 in total. An 8-channel multipipette in contrast costs well over a thousand dollars. Our purification optimization results also suggest several unexplored directions for future saliva-based nucleic acid diagnostics. The optimal NaCl concentrations were well below the theoretical limit required for purifying nucleic acids, suggesting that uncharacterized minerals or salts present in saliva are aiding nucleic acid binding to carboxylated beads.14 In addition, all saliva samples benefitted from additional TCEP, greater than previously published concentrations5. However, the degree to which they benefit and even the amount of RNA purified from different saliva samples varied. This suggests potential heterogeneity of RNase levels and/or RNA content between samples, which future saliva-based diagnostic test efforts should consider to make further improvements. We are nonetheless confident in our reported LOD, given its consistency across the wide variety of tested samples.

In summary, these new SARS-CoV-2 detection protocols are inexpensive, less than \$5 per test without considering labor and sample pooling, and offer improved scalability over existing tests without sacrificing sensitivity. They are especially suited for workplaces or schools with modest numbers of employees and students, from single digits to the low thousands. The minimal equipment requirements and low cost also make them well-suited for low resource environments, which still might be able to mount a medium complexity Clinical Laboratory Improvement Amendments (CLIA) lab. We note in this context that low-resource and underserved environments have been disproportionately vulnerable to the spread of SARS-CoV-2.15

REFERENCES

1. Zhu, N. *et al.* A Novel Coronavirus from Patients with Pneumonia in China, 2019. *New Engl J Med* **382**, 727–733 (2020).
2. Notomi, T. *et al.* Loop-mediated isothermal amplification of DNA. *Nucleic Acids Res* **28**, e63– e63 (2000).
3. Mori, Y., Nagamine, K., Tomita, N. & Notomi, T. Detection of Loop-Mediated Isothermal Amplification Reaction by Turbidity Derived from Magnesium Pyrophosphate Formation. *Biochem Bioph Res Co* **289**, 150–154 (2001).
4. Zhang, Y. *et al.* Enhancing colorimetric loop-mediated isothermal amplification speed and sensitivity with guanidine chloride. *Biotechniques* **69**, 178–185 (2020).
5. Rabe, B. A. & Cepko, C. SARS-CoV-2 detection using isothermal amplification and a rapid, inexpensive protocol for sample inactivation and purification. *Proc National Acad Sci* **117**, 24450–24458 (2020).
6. Thi, V. L. D. *et al.* A colorimetric RT-LAMP assay and LAMP-sequencing for detecting SARS-CoV-2 RNA in clinical samples. *Sci Transl Med* **12**, eabc7075 (2020).
7. Lalli, M. A. *et al.* Rapid and extraction-free detection of SARS-CoV-2 from saliva with colorimetric LAMP. *Medrxiv* 2020.05.07.20093542 (2020) doi:10.1101/2020.05.07.20093542.
8. Zhang, Y. *et al.* Rapid Molecular Detection of SARS-CoV-2 (COVID-19) Virus RNA Using Colorimetric LAMP. *Medrxiv* 2020.02.26.20028373 (2020) doi:10.1101/2020.02.26.20028373.
9. Thi, V. L. D. *et al.* Screening for SARS-CoV-2 infections with colorimetric RT-LAMP and LAMP sequencing. *Medrxiv* 2020.05.05.20092288 (2020) doi:10.1101/2020.05.05.20092288.
10. Grimm, J. B., Brown, T. A., Tkachuk, A. N. & Lavis, L. D. General Synthetic Method for Si- Fluoresceins and Si-Rhodamines. *Acs Central Sci* **3**, 975–985 (2017).
11. Wyllie, A. L. *et al.* Saliva or Nasopharyngeal Swab Specimens for Detection of SARS-CoV- 2. *New Engl J Med* **383**, 1283–1286 (2020).
12. Rohland, N. & Reich, D. Cost-effective, high-throughput DNA sequencing libraries for multiplexed target capture. *Genome Res* **22**, 939–946 (2012).
13. Kellner, M. J. *et al.* A rapid, highly sensitive and open-access SARS-CoV-2 detection assay for laboratory
14. and home testing. *Biorxiv* 2020.06.23.166397 (2020) doi:10.1101/2020.06.23.166397
15. Lis, J. T. & Schleif, R. Size fractionation of double-stranded DNA by precipitation with polyethylene glycol. *Nucleic Acids Res* **2**, 383–390 (1975).
16. Wang, M. L. *et al.* Addressing inequities in COVID-19 morbidity and mortality: research and policy recommendations. *Transl Behav Med* **10**, 516–519 (2020).

FIGURES AND FIGURE LEGENDS

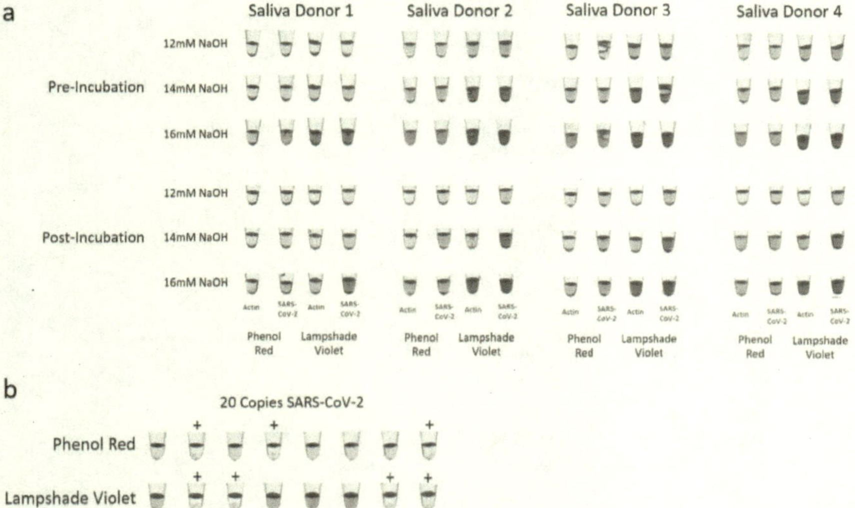

Figure 1. Two comparisons of Phenol Red against LAMPShade Violet for detection of amplification products in RT-LAMP.

(a) A comparison of color change fidelity and consistency before and after incubation in four varied saliva samples as a function of NaOH.

(b) A comparison of the sensitivity of the commercial Phenol Red RT-LAMP mix and our in-house reaction mix with LAMPShade Violet judged by their ability to detect 20 total copies of SARS- CoV-2 RNA.

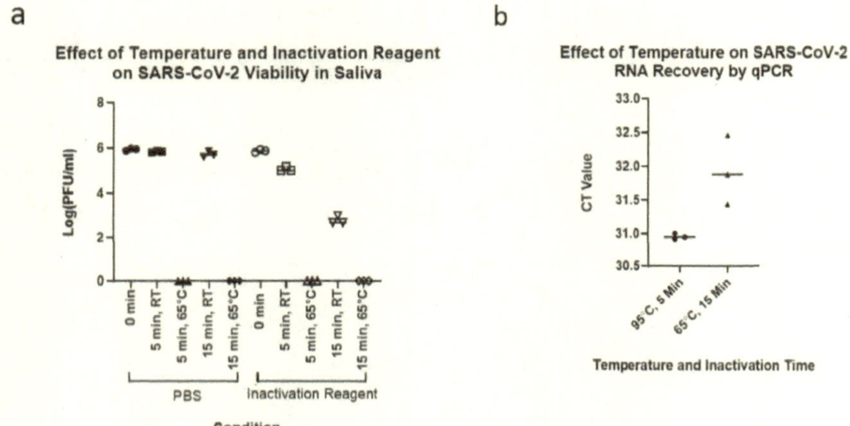

Figure 2. Evaluation of inactivation of saliva samples at 65C.

(a) A comparison of room temperature and 65C incubations on the viability of SARS-CoV-2 infected Vero E-6 cells with or without inactivation reagent.

(b) A comparison of RNA recovery from encapsulated inactivated SARS-CoV-2 virions in saliva at 95C for 5 minutes and 65C for 10 minutes.

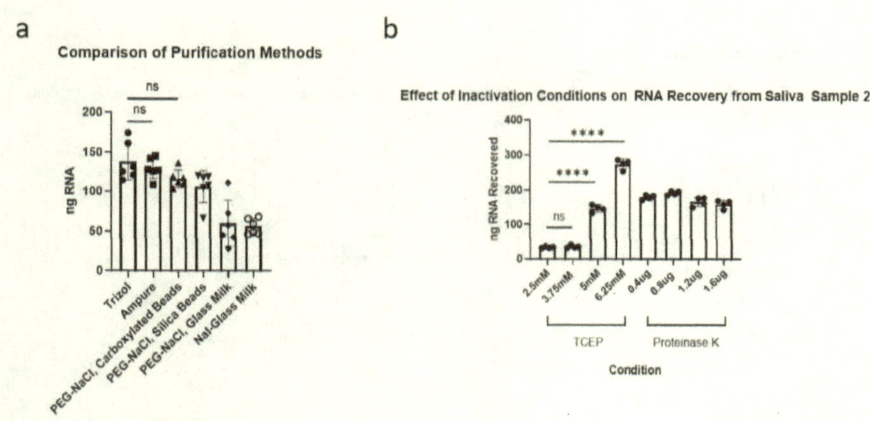

Figure 3. Investigating and optimizing saliva for purification.

(a) A comparison of select purification methods on total RNA recovered from saliva measured by Qubit fluorimetry.

(b) A comparison of RNA recovered from PEG-NaCl, Carboxylated beads following inactivation methods using different concentrations of TCEP or Proteinase K.

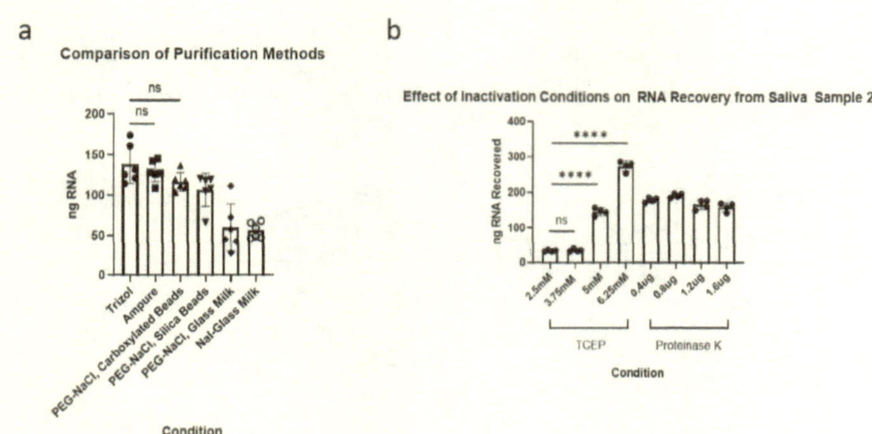

Figure 4. Optimizing the concentrations of salt and PEG for RNA purification from saliva.

(a) A Comparison of multiple salts at multiple concentrations on RNA recovery from Saliva with 18% PEG. **Top:** Measurement of recovery by Qubit fluorimetry. **Bottom:** Measurement of SARS-CoV-2 RNA recovery by N1 qCPR from contrived saliva samples.

(b) A comparison of the effect of multiple PEG concentrations with 700mM NaCl on RNA recovery, measured by SARS-CoV-2 RNA recovery by N1 qPCR from contrived saliva samples.

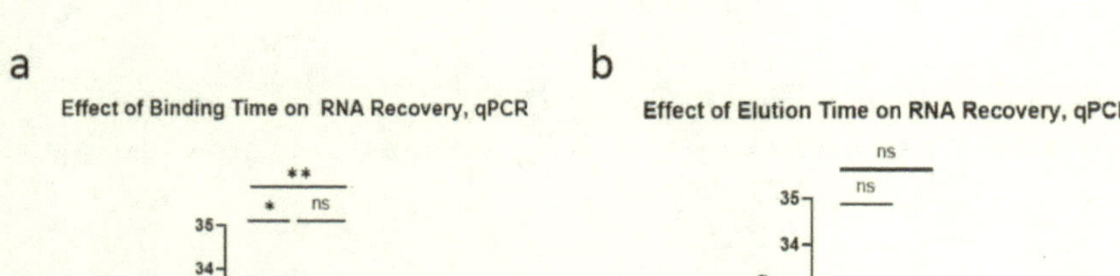

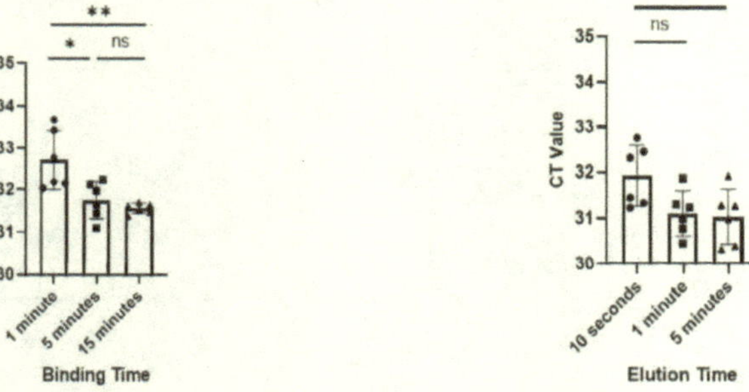

Figure 5. Optimizing the binding and elution times for magnetic bead-based purification using carboxylated beads with 700mM NaCl and 14% PEG, as measured by SARS-CoV-2 RNA recovery through N1 qPCR from contrived saliva samples.

(a) The effect of binding time on RNA recovery, with a 1-minute elution. (b) The effect of elution time on RNA recovery, with a 5-minute binding time).

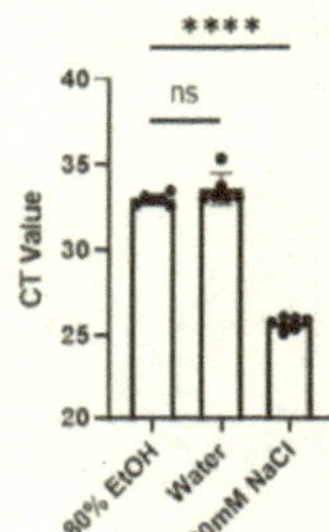

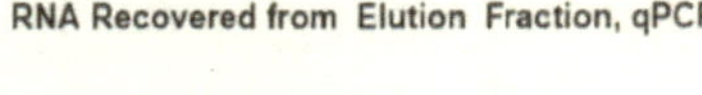

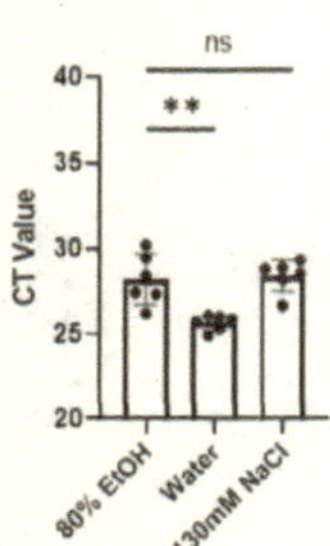

Figure 6. A comparison of three washing conditions for RNA purification from saliva using carboxylated beads with 700mM NaCl and 14% PEG, as measured by SARS-CoV-2 RNA recovery by N1 qPCR from contrived saliva samples.

(a) A measurement of RNA recovered from a 30 second wash in the indicated wash buffer.

(b) A measurement of RNA recovered from a 30 second elution in water from samples washed using the indicated wash buffer.

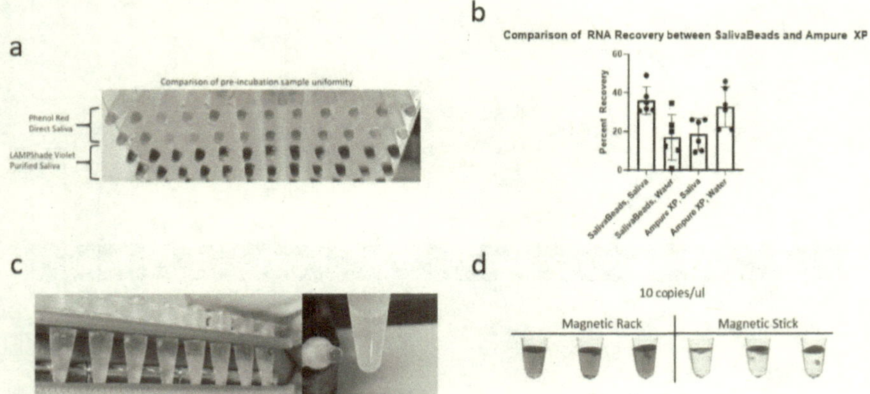

Figure 7. Several features of SalivaBeads purification.

(a) A comparison of pre-incubation sample color uniformity in 12 samples, with SARS-CoV-2 and Actin reactions side by side. Direct input of inactivated saliva in a commercial Phenol Red-based reaction is compared to a SalivaBeads-purified RNA input into our LAMPShade Violet-based reaction.

(b) A comparison of SARS-CoV-2 RNA recovered from contrived saliva samples by N1 qPCR, measured by number of copies recovered by qPCR divided by number of copies contrived into saliva.

(c) A visual comparison of debris bound to magnetic-beads when isolating beads by magnetic rack (left) or a magnetic stick (right).

(d) A comparison of sensitivity between SalivaBeads purified via magnetic rack (left) and magnetic stick (right), by RT-LAMP with LAMPShade Violet.

a

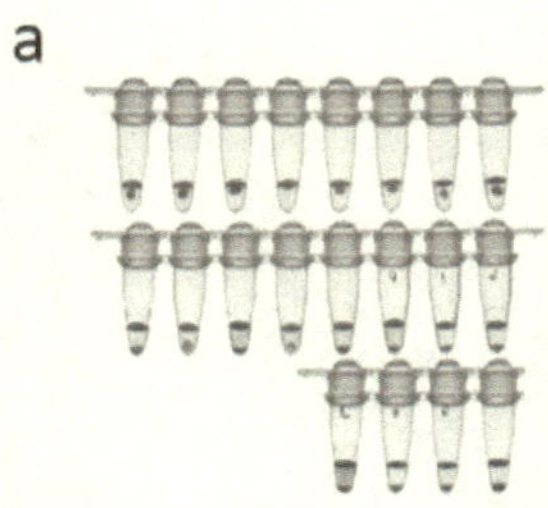

b

	3.7 copy/ul	0 copy/ul		3.7 copy/ul	0 copy/ul
Individual #1	2/2	0/2	Individual #9	2/2	0/2
Individual #2	2/2	0/2	Individual #10	2/2	0/2
Individual #3	2/2	0/2	Individual #11	2/2	0/2
Individual #4	2/2	0/2	Individual #12	3/4	0/2
Individual #5	2/2	0/2	Individual #13	2/2	0/2
Individual #6	2/2	0/2	Individual #14	2/2	0/2
Individual #7	2/2	0/2	Individual #15	2/2	0/2
Individual #8	2/2	0/2	Individual #16	2/2	0/2

Figure 8. Performance evaluation of SalivaBeads and StickLAMP.

(a) Limit of detection experiment: Ability of StickLAMP to detect 3.7 copies/µl of SARS-CoV-2 RNA from 200µl of contrived saliva in 20 replicates.

(b) Testing the ability of StickLAMP to detect 3.7 copies/µl in 200µl saliva from 16 different samples.

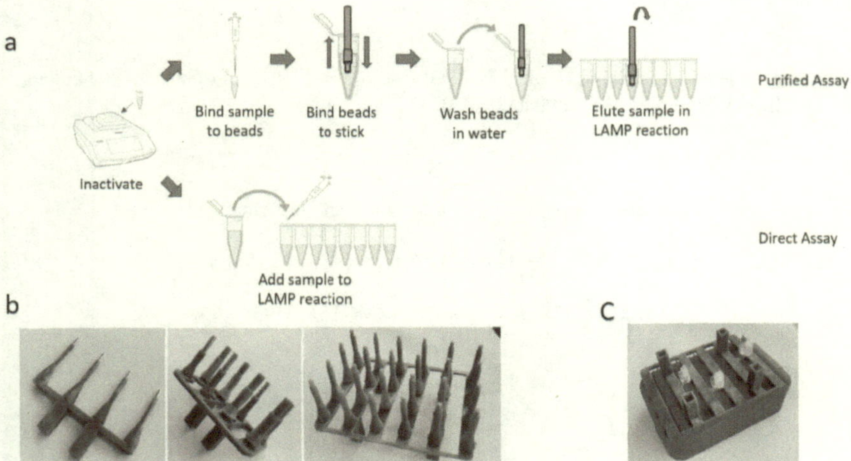

Figure 9. An overview of StickLAMP and further considerations.

(a) A visual overview of the StickLAMP protocol.

(b) A 4-channel magnetic stick (Left), 8-channel (Middle), and 24- channel (Right).

(c) A demonstration of a 24-channel magnetic stick in 3D-printed hardware designed to hold 24 1.5ml Eppendorf tubes.

CHAPTER 3

Butt-Seq: a new method for facile profiling of transcription

Albert D. Yu[1], Michael Rosbash[1*]

[1] Department of Biology, Howard Hughes Medical Institute and National Center for Behavioral Genomics, Brandeis University, Waltham, MA 02453, USA

This work has been published at Genes and Development

Genes Dev. 2023 May 1;37(9-10):432-448. doi: 10.1101/gad.350434.123. Epub 2023 May 10.

PMID: 37164645; PMCID: PMC10270195.

chromatin-associated RNA sequencing (chrRNA-seq) (Khodor et al., 2012; Sousa-Luis et al., 2021). Other techniques aim to track RNA synthesis at single-nucleotide resolution by ligating adapters to and sequencing the 3' ends of nascent RNA molecules; the logic is that the 3' end is the most recently synthesized base. These 3'end techniques include short capped RNA sequencing (scRNA-seq), 3' nucleotide sequencing (3NT-seq), and human native elongating transcript sequencing (hNET-Seq) (Mayer et al., 2015; Nechaev et al., 2010; Weber et al., 2014). scRNA-seq and 3NT-seq also feature the enrichment of capped RNA by digestion of uncapped RNA with terminator exonuclease. A variation of 3' end sequencing techniques involves the immunoprecipitation of RNAPII to enable phosphorylation-state specific profiling of nascent RNA. They include native elongating transcript sequencing (NET-Seq) and its derivatives, e.g., mammalian NET-Seq (mNET-Seq) and enhanced NET-Seq (eNET-Seq) (Churchman & Weissman, 2012; Fong et al., 2022; Nojima et al., 2015).

These powerful techniques that sequence biochemically purified nascent RNA also confront some contamination issues, for example by mature chromatin-associated RNAs like snoRNAs. Thus, care must be taken when interpreting signal. Moreover, all of these methods share two less than ideal features: the protocols are relatively complex and time-consuming, and they have quite high input material requirements.

To circumvent these features, we have devised a novel approach towards sequencing the 3'ends of biochemically purified nascent RNA, which we have named Butt-Seq (**Bu**lk analysis of nascent **t**ranscript **t**ermini sequencing). Butt-Seq leverages an optimized Thermostable Group II Intron Reverse Transcriptase (TGIRT) reverse transcription protocol to couple adapter ligation and reverse transcription into a single step (Mohr et al., 2013).

TGIRT was the first among a growing class of Group II intron reverse transcriptases that exhibits useful characteristics such as high processivity and/or thermal stability. These features have seen TGIRT employed in a variety of biochemical assays, including sequencing of highly structured RNAs such as tRNAs and small RNAs, RNA structure probing, ssDNA sequencing and others (Begik et al., 2023; Wu & Lambowitz, 2017; Xu et al., 2021; Yao et al., 2020; Zubradt et al., 2017). TGIRT is also distinguished by its ability to template switch from the 5' end of a fully reverse transcribed RNA template onto the 3' end of a new RNA template. By using an RNA/DNA hybrid primer that mimics a fully reverse transcribed RNA molecule, TGIRT can "ligate" the DNA half of the primer onto any subsequent cDNA by template switching to a target RNA molecule (Mohr et al., 2013). Typical 3'-end labeling techniques rely on T4 RNA ligase to ligate an adapter, an RNA fragmentation step, and cDNA synthesis conducted in sequential steps (Churchman & Weissman, 2012).

This Butt-Seq protocol is used for second- as well as first-strand synthesis with several other optimizations, such as a salt-concentration switching step to maximize the efficiency of the initial template switch and minimize subsequent, undesirable template switches; the protocol also uses a low concentration of dNTPs to minimize DNA fragment size. These features eliminate the need for RNA fragmentation and condenses multiple materially demanding gel extraction steps into a single post-PCR extraction step. Butt-Seq can prepare libraries from purified nascent RNA in as few as 6 hours and exhibits reproducible signal with inputs as low as 10,000 *Drosophila* S2 cells. This input requirement represents at least a 10-fold improvement over existing protocols; other NET-Seq like techniques typically reference inputs of 1,000,000-10,000,000 cells, while qPRO-Seq requires 100,000 cells (Churchman & Weissman, 2012; Judd et al., 2020; Mayer et al., 2015; Nojima et al., 2015). Butt-Seq also is effective with limited input material from biological tissue, which we demonstrate by profiling small numbers of *Drosophila* heads.

When selecting a technique to analyze nascent RNA, it is important to understand the limits of each technique. For example, 3'-end labeling is a powerful approach for resolving RNA polymerase positioning, but an increase in signal density can either reflect an increase in transcription or decrease in transcriptional elongation rate. Here we examined this ambiguity by using Butt-Seq to investigate the regulation of core circadian genes. Circadian rhythms are governed by a transcriptional feedback loop wherein the clock (*Clk*)/cycle(*cyc)* heterodimer drive the transcription of negative regulator genes period (*per)* and timeless (*tim*), which repress the activity of *Clk/cyc* and thereby downregulate their own transcription (Hardin, 2005). This feedback loop is a well-characterized paradigm driven by *de novo* transcription, so we examined the transcription of core clock genes to assess the ability of Butt-Seq to measure relative transcription rate (Rodriguez et al., 2013; So & Rosbash, 1997).

Promoter-proximal pausing is another feature of transcription that we address with Butt-Seq. Such pausing is a ubiquitous and conserved regulatory step in transcriptional regulation, wherein RNA polymerase pauses after transcribing a short stretch of RNA to await further regulatory signaling before proceeding into processive elongation (Jonkers & Lis, 2015). Pause release is dependent on phosphorylation of the RNAPII C-terminal domain (CTD) by Cyclin-dependent kinase 9 (Cdk9) as part of the positive-transcription elongation factor b (P-TEFb) complex (Jonkers & Lis, 2015; Liang et al., 2018). P-TEFb is largely sequestered in its inactive form, but its incorporation into the Super Elongation Complex (SEC) is one means by which it can be directed to drive pause release. The *Drosophila* SEC is comprised of the elongation Suppressor of Triplolethal (*Su(Tpl*), ELL-associated factor (*Eaf),* ENL/AF9-like protein (*ear)*, and the AFF (AF4/FMR2 family)-like protein Lilliputian (*lilli*) (Dahlberg et al., 2015). We treated S2 cells with the AFF4/*lilli* inhibitor KL-1 and examined the effect on pause release with Butt-Seq. Pharmaceutically inhibiting the

SEC with KL-1 causes pause sites to recede upstream in a chromatin-dependent fashion, showing that Butt-Seq can resolve RNA polymerase localization at single nucleotide resolution and implying that promoter-proximal pausing regulation may involve the clearance of multiple discrete pausing sites.

Altogether, we establish Butt-Seq as a simple and powerful method capable of resolving multiple aspects of transcription that offers several attractive improvements over existing methods.

RESULTS

Butt-Seq is an efficient 3' Nascent RNA end-labeling technique

Nascent RNA contains a heterogeneous mixture of molecules in varying states of synthesis. They include short transcripts associated with paused RNA polymerase, partially synthesized RNAs , and completed transcripts awaiting cleavage and polyadenylation (Wissink et al., 2019). Butt-Seq is inspired by other 3'-end labeling techniques and captures the entire breadth of all nascent transcripts. However, the data presented focus on transcripts from protein-coding genes.

The protocol first isolates chromatin with 0.5M Urea and 1.5% Empigen as previously described (Rodriguez et al., 2013; Schlackow et al., 2017; Sousa-Luis et al., 2021). The resulting chromatin-associated RNA undergoes simultaneous adapter ligation and reverse transcription using the TGIRT reverse transcriptase and an adapter containing the read 2 sequence. There is also an 8-bp UMI in place of the usual i7 index as well as the P7 sequence. A short reverse transcription step is conducted with a low concentration of dNTPs; this is to limit the length of the cDNA and minimize length-dependent biases when sequencing. The final insert should be no longer than 350nt in length. Furthermore, pre-RT incubation is done with a low concentration of salt, while dNTPs are added along with a higher concentration of salt; this is done to maximize the efficiency of the initial template switch, but to minimize the amount of secondary template switches as well as slow down reverse transcription. Second-strand synthesis and Read 1 adaptor ligation are conducted through a second TGIRT reaction, and the final adapter-tagged cDNA is subject to PCR with standard i5 indexing primer, gel extraction, and standard Illumina sequencing. The resulting library should reflect all chromatin-associated RNA, most notably a high-resolution view of polymerase pausing and transcriptional elongation (Figure 1A).

Butt-Seq results are comparable to those from other established methods

A major use of 3'-end labeling techniques is the identification and characterization of promoter-proximal pausing, represented by regions of distinctly high signal adjacent to the transcription start site (Mayer et al., 2017). Such pausing represents a distinct regulatory step: RNAPII transcribes a short stretch of RNA before pausing and awaiting further signaling before either disengaging or proceeding into processive elongation. To validate Butt-Seq for pausing analysis, we examined the average signal distribution 200nt downstream of the TSS genome-wide in *Drosophila* S2 cells and compared it to the signal from published data in these cells generated by other nascent RNA techniques: 3NT-Seq, PRO-Seq, and RNAPII ChIP-Seq (Figure 1B). All four techniques feature a sharp peak directly downstream of the TSS, likely driven by the high prevalence of promoter-proximal pausing across the genome, followed by signal reflecting transcripts undergoing processive elongation.

We quantified these regions and performed a log-log comparison of Butt-Seq against the three published techniques. Butt-Seq has the highest correlation to the most chemically analogous technique, 3NT-Seq (Spearman correlation = 0.73), but also correlates well with RNAPII ChIP-Seq (Spearman's correlation = 0.67) and PRO-Seq (Spearman's correlation = 0.59). These relationships apply similarly to the gene body, where Butt-Seq also correlates well with 3NT-Seq (Spearman's correlation = 0.71), PRO-Seq (Spearman's correlation = 0.69), and RNAPII ChIP-Seq (Spearman's correlation = 0.71). These comparisons indicate that Butt-Seq faithfully assays nascent RNA.

One point of concern in 3' end labeling techniques is the presence of small RNA and/or rRNA contaminants, which can drive up experimental costs by increasing the amount of required sequencing depth. 3NT-Seq incorporates a terminator exonuclease step to degrade uncapped RNA species to reduce the number of undesirable analytes (Weber et al., 2014); Butt-Seq forgoes this step. Nonetheless, the extent of small RNA and rRNA contamination is similar between the two techniques (Supplemental Fig. S1A and S1B). As expected, PRO-Seq exhibits virtually no small RNA contamination and approximately 15% less rRNA contamination. In any case, Butt-Seq produces data of comparable quality to existing techniques in its class. As with other 3'-end labeling techniques, small RNAs and other contaminants are removed computationally prior to downstream analyses.

Butt-Seq is reproducible down to 10,000 cells

We next assayed the minimum input requirement for Butt-Seq. Our eventual goal is to assay primary tissues or cells from which material may be limited. The Butt-Seq signal 200nt downstream of the TSS correlated well between 500,000 and 50,000 cells (Spearman's correlation = 0.97), and even between 500,000 and 10,000 cells (Spearman's correlation = 0.91) (Figure 2A). There is a similar signal distribution pattern: all feature a sharp peak at the TSS indicative of promoter-proximal pausing (Figure 2B). The high correlation coefficients indicates that Butt-Seq is not only highly reproducible but also consistent with 10,000 cells or less.

KL-1 causes pause sites to recede towards the TSS

We next used Butt-Seq to characterize the effect of the AFF4/lilliputian (*lilli*) inhibitor, KL-1, on transcription in S2 cells. KL-1 disrupts the formation of the superelongation complex (SEC) by inhibiting *lilli* activity (Liang et al., 2018). It thereby impedes the release of paused polymerase into productive elongation and attenuates the rate of elongation. As KL-1 has previously been shown to result in an increased RNAPII ChIP-Seq signal at the TSS, we compared Butt-Seq signal to published RNAPII ChIP-Seq data (Liang et al., 2018).

To assay the genome-wide pausing index of 20μM KL-1-treated S2 cells compared to vehicle

(DMSO)-treated cells, we calculated the signal ratio between promoter-adjacent reads and gene body reads (Figure 3A). Pausing index is usually calculated by dividing the signal in a fixed TSS adjacent region by the signal in the gene body. The TSS adjacent region is typically defined as the -50 region to the +300 region, although this can vary from study to study (Liang et al., 2018). While this definition has been employed to great effect in ChIP-Seq studies, single-nucleotide resolution techniques enable more precision. We used a novel peak-calling algorithm developed for single-nucleotide techniques – the Pause Detection Algorithm (PDA) – to detect pauses in the first 200 bases downstream of the TSS (Gajos et al., 2021). We then filtered pauses to find the highest signal, so that each gene only has a single pause site. We then analyzed pause sites detected by PDA for motifs and identified an enrichment of G/A and T/C residues at the -1 and +1 nucleotide, respectively, similar to previously reported motifs (Supplemental Fig. S2A). The enriched motifs further indicate that these are proper pause sites, and we therefore defined the pausing region as extending from the TSS to the pause site, and the gene body as the region 2kb downstream of the pause site. By measuring the pausing index on an Empirical Cumulative Distribution Function (ECDF) plot, there was a significant increase in pausing index upon KL-1 treatment (Kolmogorov-Smirnov, $D = 0.11815$, $p < 2.2e-16$), as had been previously reported in RNAPII ChIP-Seq data (Figure 3A) (Liang et al., 2018). We also calculated the pausing index using the standard method. It revealed the same degree of change albeit at a lower magnitude (Kolmogorov-Smirnov, $D = 0.0424$, $p < 0.001$) (Supplemental Fig. S2A).

To analyze transcriptional dynamics at single nucleotide resolution, each Butt-Seq read was truncated to the first base sequenced by Read 2; this should reflect the last nascent RNA base synthesized by RNAPII. Surprisingly, this single-nucleotide resolution indicated that KL-1 not only increased the magnitude of pausing as previously reported but also caused genome-wide pause sites to move upstream toward the TSS (Liang et al., 2018). (A representative gene is shown in Figure 3B.) Reanalysis of published RNAPII ChIP-Seq data and metagene profiling of this RNAPII ChIP-Seq signal indicate that both conclusions are visible in these previous data (Figure 3C). First, the Butt-Seq signal peaks align with the RNAPII ChIP-Seq peaks, both for DMSO and KL-1 treated conditions. Second, treatment with KL-1 causes the signal to move in the 5' direction towards the TSS while also increasing in magnitude, suggestive of increased pausing in addition to altering the precise pause sites (Figure 3C). This effect is most pronounced in Butt-Seq, although it is also visible at lower resolution in the RNAPII ChIP-Seq data.

RNAPII positioning and KL-1 sensitivity correlate with subnucleosomal structures of the -1 nucleosome

We leveraged the single nucleotide sensitivity of Butt-Seq to address the relationship between RNAPII pausing and subnucleosome structure. MNase-seq is used to measure nucleosome positioning, and selective sequencing and analysis of sub-nucleosomal (<147bp) MNase-digested fragments can be used to map partially unwrapped subnucleosomal particles (Ramachandran et al., 2017). We therefore examined the relationship of the Butt-Seq signals to previously published subnucleosomal MNase-seq data from S2 cells (Ramachandran et al., 2017). These fragments typically exhibit a bimodal distribution, representing protection from digestion by the two halves of a partially unwrapped histone dyad (Visible in Figure 4A, top). RNAPII proximity to the +1 nucleosome correlates with loss of the dyad distal to the TSS (Ramachandran et al., 2017). This observation was inferred to be a causal result of RNAPII transcribing through the nucleosome. However, many studies suggest the opposite: even the subnucleosome particle is a transcriptional barrier capable of slowing and pausing RNAPII, which then can be overcome by RNAPII through a number of molecular strategies. In any case, we asked whether subnucleosomal dynamics correlate with KL-1 sensitivity.

We first measured the genome-wide distribution of the Butt-Seq signal and the MNase-Seq signal restricted to 58 +/- 5 bp fragments (Figure 4A). A surprising number of MNase peaks with a bimodal distribution overlapped the TSS (N=1684) (visible in Figure 4A, top). The region overlapping the TSS is typically thought to be a nucleosome free-region, and the -1 nucleosome is defined as the region just preceding the TSS. However, this 58bp pattern is consistent with protection by a subnucleosomal H3-H4 dyad, a distribution referred to as a -1 nucleosome (Ramachandran et al., 2017); we will use this terminology. Pausing was enriched in genes exhibiting this fragment distribution pattern and was also sensitive to KL-1 treatment (Figure 4A, bottom). In contrast, pausing was depleted in genes enriched with the H2Av variant in the +1 nucleosome as previously shown (Figure 4B)(Weber et al., 2014). Surprisingly however, H2Av-enriched genes were also sensitive to KL-1 treatment.

To further analyze these Butt-Seq pause sites, we divided them into 5 clusters based on their distance downstream from the center of the -1 nucleosome (Figure 4C). Cluster 1 contains pauses 80-120bp downstream of the -1 nucleosome, Cluster 2 contains pauses 60-79bp downstream, Cluster 3 contains pauses 40-59bp downstream, Cluster 4 contains pauses 20-39 downstream, while Cluster 5 contains pauses 0-19 bases downstream. To examine the relationship between the pausing clusters, KL-1 sensitivity and nucleosome occupancy, we plotted MNase-Seq and KL-1 treated Butt-Seq signals against the DMSO-treated signal in each cluster; this revealed two notable patterns (Figure 4D).

First, the character of the nucleosome dyad changes in each cluster. In Cluster 1, where the pause site is furthest from the -1 nucleosome, both halves of the nucleosomal dyad are present. In Cluster 5, where the pause site is very close to the +1 nucleosome, the distal half of the nucleosome dyad is completely absent. Moving from Cluster 1 to Cluster 5, there is a gradual loss of the nucleosome dyad distal half (Figure 4D, blue). Second, the effect of KL-1 treatment on the pause site appears to be impacted by the distance of the pause site to the nucleosome center; the further downstream the pause site, the greater the effect of KL-1.

Butt-Seq identifies differential pausing dynamics between S2 cells and *Drosophila* heads

In contrast to the extensive amount of research conducted on tissue-specific gene expression programs, tissue-specific pausing has received rather little attention (Day et al., 2016). The extent to which an identically expressed set of genes may be differentially regulated by pausing is therefore poorly understood. One of the primary advantages of Butt-Seq is that its more relaxed input material requirements enable a more facile profiling of primary tissues. To exploit this feature, Butt-Seq was used to profile nascent RNA from a small number (n = 5) Canton-S *Drosophila* heads and compared to the S2 cell profiles. These two very different tissues are not surprisingly poorly correlated (Spearman's correlation = 0.30) (Figure 5A). However, many commonly expressed genes have similar single-nucleotide pausing signatures (Figure 5B).

We sought to explore the extent to which transcriptional programs might vary between the two tissues. For example, are there genes commonly expressed between the two tissues, but elongation in only one tissue is gated by a pause-release step? To further explore the variation in pausing and elongation dynamics between heads and S2 cells, we first called single-nucleotide peaks separately from S2 cells and heads, restricting the peak calling to within 200nt of the TSS and filtering for the highest signal when a gene had multiple peaks. We then merged peaks between S2 cells and heads and compared signals in pausing regions and elongation regions of each gene: We defined the pause region as the region between the pause peak and the TSS and the elongation region as a gene body region 1000bp downstream of the pause peak. We then compared the relative signal between the pause region and the elongation region between S2 cells and heads (Figure 6).

Pausing and elongation are concordant in 61% of genes; when pausing is higher in one tissue, elongation is also higher, and vice versa (Figure 6A top, Figure 6B and 6C middle, 6D). These genes might simply manifest tissue differences in rates of transcriptional initiation. In most of the other genes (31%), there was a discordant relationship between pause and elongation regions: heads and S2 cells exhibit the same signal in one parameter, but a different signal in the other (Figure 6B and 6C, top and bottom). Most notably, 8% of genes are discordant for both parameters, e.g., when pausing is higher in one tissue, elongation is lower. These genes may therefore experience differential bottlenecking by pause release factors, suggesting the presence of different transcriptional programs regulating commonly expressed genes.

Butt-Seq identifies transcriptional dynamics in key circadian genes

We and others have previously measured the association of RNAPII with circadian clock genes in fly heads at different times of day (Abruzzi et al., 2011), for example by ChIP-Seq. Taken together with other assays (Taylor & Hardin, 2008), there is strong evidence that RNAPII cycles on and off clock gene chromatin in gene body regions in a circadian manner and parallels cycling clock gene transcription. There is however one striking exception: there are substantial levels of RNAPII stably associated with the *period (per)* gene promoter region at all times of day, even at times of day when there is little transcription (Abruzzi et al., 2011; Taylor & Hardin, 2008). Will Butt-Seq recapitulate or perhaps even extend these previous observations? To answer this question, we assayed fly head nuclei from entrained flies collected at 6 times of day, ZT2-ZT22 (ZT is time in a 12:12 LD cycle, with ZT0=lights on and ZT12=lights off).

As anticipated, the clock gene body signal undergoes robust circadian cycling with peaks at ZT14 and troughs at ZT2 for the CLK/CYC direct target genes *per, vri* and *tim,* and a peak at ZT2 and a trough at ZT14 for the clock gene *Clk.* (Figure 6). Notably, the *per* Butt-Seq data show a prominent and stable signal across peak and trough timepoints just downstream of the transcription start site (Figure 7A top left). This indicates that pause release might be under circadian regulation and contribute to *per* transcription. In contrast, the other two direct target genes *vri* and *tim* differ from *per.* Although *tim* and *vri* show notable pause sites near their TSSs (Figure 7A top right and bottom left), they oscillate with a similar amplitude to the gene body (Figure 7A and data not shown). This suggests that the transcription of these 2 genes is primarily regulated through oscillating transcription initiation. The *Clk* gene in contrast features a much smaller but temporally constant pause site like that of *per*, which implies that *Clk* may also be at least partially regulated through pause release.

Butt-Seq recapitulates circadian transcriptional oscillation details

Could Butt-Seq be used to assess different transcription rates? Although a high Butt-Seq signal in gene body regions may reflect a high level of RNA production, it may also reflect a high level of RNAPII occupancy due to a slow rate of transcriptional elongation. However, both NET-seq and RNAPII ChIP-Seq signal have previously been used to approximate transcription levels of RNA synthesis, which is because RNAPII occupancy often if not usually reflects RNA synthesis. To examine in quantitative detail this putative circadian transcriptional regulation, we calculated the Butt-Seq signal within every gene at each of the six time points; only exon signals were summed, i.e., intron signals were removed to avoid possible complications from nascent splicing. To help interpret the data, we turned to two published head time point mRNA-seq datasets - one generated by our lab almost 10 years ago and the other generated elsewhere five years ago (Kuintzle et al., 2017; Rodriguez et al., 2013). For ease of illustration, we focus here on the four core clock direct CLK-target genes presented above (Figure 7A) and double plotted these two data sets along with our Butt-Seq data (Figure 7B).

A first notable observation is that the two RNA-seq data sets are very similar; the *tim* and *vri* curves are indistinguishable, whereas only the peak values of the *Clk* profiles and to a lesser extent the *per* profiles are somewhat different (Figure 7B, purple and blue). A second is that the Butt-Seq data are virtually superimposable onto the RNA-seq data for 3 of the four genes. This suggests that transcriptional regulation accounts for almost all mRNA dynamics for these four core clock genes (Figure 7B).

The only notable exception is *per*. The Butt-Seq data indicate that the mid-day increase in transcription is phase-advanced relative to the RNA-seq data. Because the nighttime decreases are coincident, this makes for a broader Butt-Seq plateau between ZT10 and ZT14 relative to the RNA-seq data (Figure 7B; green arrows). Remarkably, this comparison is identical to what we reported in a comparison between a nuclear run-on assay of per transcription and a RNase protection assay of steady-state per mRNA (So & Rosbash, 1997). Those assays were low throughput, limiting the number of genes that could be examined. Nonetheless, *tim* was assessed in parallel and was more equivocal, i.e., it did not show such a striking distinction between transcription and mRNA levels (So & Rosbash, 1997); this is similar to what we observe here between tim Butt-Seq and RNA-seq data (Figure 7B). The parallels between these two different assays done twenty-five years apart indicate that the circadian regulation of *per* is quantitatively and perhaps even qualitatively unusual compared to the other core clock genes and most importantly support the assertion that the Butt-Seq exon signal successfully assays transcription.

DISCUSSION

Butt-Seq is a facile method for the analysis of nascent RNA and sequences the 3'-ends of chromatin associated RNA. In most analyzed reads, the 3' end is the base most recently synthesized by RNAPII. Although this same strategy is employed by a wide range of methods, Butt-Seq offers a much simpler workflow: it can produce libraries from purified nascent RNA in as few as six hours and is reproducible down to 10,000 cells.

Although the choice of TGIRT for reverse transcription and adaptor ligation is the most notable difference from these previous methods, many of them employ selection steps that Butt-seq does not, for example phosphorylation-state specific immunoprecipitation of RNAPII. scRNA-seq and 3NT-seq also deplete uncapped RNA species with a cap-sensitive exonuclease. Although Butt-Seq circumvents this step, it nevertheless correlates well with 3NT-Seq (Figure 1B and 1C), suggesting that cap-selection may not have a large effect on signal in regions of interest. Relative to these earlier methods, Butt-seq bears the greatest resemblance to hNET-seq, which also does not incorporate a selection step. Despite the lack of a polymerase-bound or capped RNA selection in the Butt-Seq protocol, it shows similar signals at protein-coding genes with a much simplified workflow and improved input requirements.

The capacity of Butt-Seq to address transcriptional pausing detail is highlighted in experiments demonstrating that the transcriptional elongation and SEC inhibitor KL-1 causes transcriptional pause sites to recede towards the TSS. The extent of this movement was relatively short – approximately 10 to 80 base pairs – making the possibility that this change in signal is due to changes in TSS selection unlikely. Furthermore, we did not observe widespread TSS selection changes upon KL-1 treatment. This observation implies the existence of multiple pausing checkpoints downstream from the TSS, the closest of which is rapidly resolved by the recruitment of the SEC shortly after transcriptional initiation. The existence of multiple pausing checkpoints resembles the recently proposed "pausing zone," a region of enhanced RNA polymerase pausing adjacent to the transcription start site (Fong et al., 2022). Notably, this paper reported that a phosphorylation mutant of Spt5 – Spt5 KOWx4-KOW5 – exhibited increased signal density in regions of the pausing zone adjacent to the TSS, suggesting that this phosphorylation mutant impedes the ability of RNAPII to exit this early pausing zone. This pausing zone finding corroborates our observation of multiple pause sites and suggests that this mode of pause-release regulation may be conserved between insects and mammals. Unlike the study focused on the KOWx4-KOW5 mutant however, we focused our analysis on the shifting of discrete major pause sites. In addition, close examination of the metagene plots suggests that KL-1 treatment causes increased signal at least 500bp into the gene body, which hints that a pausing zone exists in our data as well.

These pause sites have an intriguing relationship to subnucleosomal fragments obtained through MNase-Seq: increased proximity of the pause site to the -1 nucleosome center is negatively correlated with sensitivity to KL-1 treatment and positively correlated with a loss of contact with the distal half of the nucleosomal dyad. These differences in nucleosomal contacts may be a consequence of RNAPII proximity as previously suggested(Ramachandran et al., 2017). However, the insensitivity to KL-1 in genes with pause sites directly adjacent to the center of the nucleosome suggests more complex regulation. Surprisingly, KL-1 appears to also cause transcriptional deceleration near the TSS in genes containing H2Av in the +1 nucleosome, which is depleted of promoter-proximal pausing in *Drosophila*(Weber et al., 2014). This suggests that recruitment of the SEC might occur concurrently with transcriptional initiation at H2Av-marked genes, which then bypasses promoter-proximal pausing.

A strength of Butt-Seq should be its ability to interrogate samples where input material may be limited, like primary tissue. To this end, we assayed fly heads with Butt-Seq at 6 different timepoints and focused on 4 clock genes. *per* features a very prominent stable pause signal as previously observed. Future experiments should indicate whether the rhythmic transcription of *per* is regulated at least in part through pause release. In this context, there is evidence that *per* mRNA is more stable early in its accumulation cycle (So et al.). This is when pause release should be prominent, before the large RNAPII increase in the elongating region. Perhaps there is a mRNP difference between transcripts due to pause release compared to those that accumulate later due to increased transcriptional initiation.

In this context, we have previously explored the relative contributions of transcriptional vs. post-transcriptional regulation to circadian mRNA oscillations. Given that the Butt-Seq signal along the gene body represents an uncommon approach towards examining transcriptional dynamics – essentially, the quantification of RNAPII density – we revisited this question in a simple way by examining the relationship between Butt-Seq signal and mRNA-Seq signal. Interestingly, the amplitude, period, and phase of the Butt-Seq signal and the mRNA-seq signal were remarkably similar – with Butt-Seq phase leading mRNA-Seq by no more than ~1 hour. A genome-wide analysis of oscillating transcription suggests that aspects of this relationship may be general (data not shown); however, the complexity of this analysis puts it outside the scope of this methods paper. We therefore chose to focus on the core circadian clock components whose transcriptional regulation have been well characterized over decades and multiple biochemical approaches. In one previous study using nuclear run-on and RNA radiolabeling methods, we reported a "hump" of *per* transcription that precedes the peak of per mRNA; comparing the two curves suggested interesting *per* post-transcriptional regulation in addition to its more expected transcriptional regulation (So & Rosbash, 1997). The same "hump" is visible in Butt-Seq now 25 years later (Figure 6B). Although further exploration is beyond the scope of this study, these observations as well as the paused polymerase peak in the *per* promoter region (Figure 6A and Abruzzi et al. 2013(Taylor & Hardin, 2008)) suggest that *per* is subject to unusual modes of regulation relative to other Clk-regulated core circadian genes.

The extent of tissue-specific transcriptional pausing and pause release has received relatively little attention. The relationship between pausing and elongation was non-linear in differentially expressed genes between heads and S2 cells; in other words, differences in pausing signal was frequently not accompanied by a concordant change in gene body signal. This finding echoes a previous study analyzing pausing through RNAPII ChIP-Seq in different mammalian tissues (Day et al., 2016). One possibility is that pausing enables a second layer of regulation, wherein the combinatorial recruitment of initiation and pause release factors enable tissue-specific gene expression (Adelman & Lis, 2012). This discordant relationship implies that pause release may be a rate-limiting step in the expression of many genes including *per*, and that interesting tissue-specific factors may be required to enable pause-release and the transition from pausing to processive elongation. In any case, we suggest the Butt-Seq will provide future insights into transcriptional regulation from many other areas of investigation well beyond flies and circadian biology.

METHODS

S2 cell culture and KL-1 treatment

S2 cells were obtained from the ATCC (CRL-1963) and cultured in Schneiders Medium supplemented with 10% FetalGro (rmbio, FGX-BBT) and 1% Penicillin/Streptomycin (ThermoFisher, 15140122). For KL-1 treatment, S2 cells were plated in 6-well plates at a density of $1x10^6$ cells per well and left for one day. KL-1 to a final concentration of 20μM or an equal volume of DMSO was added to the cells and treated for 6 hours. Cells were harvested after 6 hours.

Nascent RNA isolation in S2 cells

Nascent RNA isolation was adapted from (Khodor et al., 2012). S2 cells grown in a T25 flask were harvested by scraping and pelleted in a centrifuge at 900g for 5 minutes, washing once with 10ml 1x cold PBS. Unless otherwise specified, $5x10^5$ cells were used. Washed cells were resuspended in 500μl cell lysis buffer (10mM Tris pH7.5, 2mM $MgCl_2$, 10mM kCl, 0.6mM spermidine, 0.2mM spermine, 3mM TCEP, 0.03% Tween-20, and 0.1% BSA) and transferred into 2ml dounce homogenizers. Cells were homogenized with 10 strokes with Pestle A and 15 strokes with Pestle B. Homogenized cells were passed through a 10μM filter (Sysmex, 04-0042-2314) and centrifuged at 1000g for 5 minutes. Supernatant was removed and nuclei were resuspended in 100μl nuclear lysis buffer (10mM HEPES-KOH pH7.6, 100mM KCl, 0.1mM EDTA, 10% Glycerol, 0.15mM Spermine, 0.5mM Spermidine, 0.1mM NaF, 0.1mM Na_3VO_4, 0.1mM $ZnCl_2$, 1mM TCEP, 0.1 units/μl SUPERaseIn, and 1x cOmplete protease inhibitor) and placed on a Thermomix set to 4°C and shaking at 1400 RPM. 100μl NUN buffer (25mM HEPES-KOH, pH7.6, 300mM NaCl, 1M Urea, 1% NP-40, 1mM TCEP, 3% Empigen, 0.1 units/μl SUPERaseIn, 1x cOmplete protease inhibitor) was added dropwise while shaking. Tubes were capped and left shaking at 4°C for 10 minutes. Chromatin was pelleted in the centrifuge at 21000g for 10 minutes, and the supernatant was discarded. The resulting chromatin pellet was resuspended in 500μl TRIzol and incubated at 60°C for 10 minutes, then transferred to a phase lock tube. RNA was then isolated with chloroform according to standard procedure and resuspended in a 10μl Turbo DNAse reaction containing 1x Turbo DNase Buffer and 1.5μl Turbo DNase, and DNase treatment was done for 30 minutes according to protocol. 2μl DNase treated RNA was used for Butt-Seq.

Nascent RNA isolation in fly heads

Flies were frozen on dry ice. 5 heads were removed on dry ice and transferred into a 2ml dounce homogenizer. 500μl nuclear lysis buffer was added to each homogenizer, and heads were dounced for 10 strokes with Pestle A and 20 strokes with Pestle B. The resulting homogenate was first filtered through a 20μM filter, then a 20μM filter. Nuclei were spun down for 1000g for 5 minutes and washed once with 500μl nuclear lysis buffer. Resulting nuclei were subject to chromatin isolation as with S2 cells.

Butt-Seq library prep

Butt-Seq library prep consists of two consecutive TGIRT protocols for first and second strand synthesis. For a detailed protocol, along with notes and rationale, please see the supplementary protocol. The first strand synthesis primer contains the read 2 sequencing primer, and UMI sequence, and the P7 sequence. The second strand synthesis primer contains only the read 1 sequencing primer. An i5 barcode and the P5 sequence are added through PCR (Figure 1A).

RNA/DNA hybrid primer assembly is similar to the commercial protocol, but with concentrations modified to reduce the volume of primer required in the reaction. Please see supplementary table for a complete table of primers used. To prepare SCR2R primer, 10μl 10μM R2 RNA (rArArGrArUrCrGrGrArArGrArGrCrArCrArCrGrUrCrUrGrArArCrUrCrCrArGrUrCrArC/3Sp C3/) was mixed with 10μl 10μM SCR2 DNA

(CAAGCAGAAGACGGCATACGAGATNNNNNNNNGTGACTGGAGTTCAGACGTGTGC TCTTCCGATCTTN), where N is a hand-mixed equimolar ratio of A/T/C/G, along with 5µl 10x annealing buffer (10mM Tris-HCl, pH7.5, 10mM EDTA, 10mM TCEP pH 7.5) and 25µl H_2O. SCR2R primer was ordered as PAGE-purified, while SCR2 DNA was ordered as a PAGE-purified Ultramer from IDT. Primers were added to a pre-heated 88°C thermal cycler, incubated for 2 minutes, and then cooled to 10°C at a rate of 0.1°C/second and held at 10°C.

To prepare MER1R primer, 10µl 10µM R1ME RNA (rCrUrGrUrCrUrCrUrUrArUrArCrArCrArUrCrUrGrArCrGrCrUrGrC/3SpC3/) was mixed with 10µl 10µM R1ME DNA (GCAGCGTCAGATGTGTATAAGAGACAGN), where N is a hand-mixed equimolar ratio of A/T/C/G, along with 5µl 10x annealing buffer (10mM Tris-HCl, pH7.5, 10mM EDTA, 10mM TCEP pH 7.5) and 25µl H_2O (Rhee & Burke, 2004). Both primers were PAGE-purified from IDT. Primers were added to a pre-heated 88°C thermal cycler, incubated for 2 minutes, and then cooled to 10°C at a rate of 0.1°C/second and held at 10°C.

All primers were aliquoted into single-used aliquots and stored at -80°C for up to 6 months.

First strand master mixes (FS-MM) were prepared with 0.5µl 10x ButtRT Buffer(100mM HEPES pH8, 500mM NaCl, 50mM $MgCl_2$, 10mM TCEP), 0.2µl SCR2R, 0.2µl TGIRT, and 1.1µl 50% PEG3350). FS-MM was prepared for at least 4 reactions at a time to minimize pipetting errors. To ensure the reactions were well-mixed, reactions were stirred ten times with a pipette tip, and flicked and spun down twice. 2µl of FS-MM was added to 2µl RNA in a PCR strip tube, flicking and spinning down twice to mix. RNA inputs between 0.5pg to 25ng have been tested, but when working with <500,000 cells, we do not quantify RNA prior to assembling the reaction. Assembled reactions were incubated on ice for 30 minutes.

While incubating, 1µl 5mM dNTPs was mixed with 30µl 2M NaCl. After 30 minutes, 1µl dNTPs/NaCl mixture was added to TGIRT reactions and placed on the thermal cycler with the following program: 25°C for 1 minute, ramping to 60°C at 1°C/second, 60°C for 10 seconds, then holding at 4°C. Reactions were moved on to ice and 2µl Exonuclease III, 2µl H_2O, and 1µl NEBuffer 1 were added and flicked to mix. Reactions were incubated at 37°C for 8 minutes, then moved onto ice. Exonuclease III treatment partially digests unused primers. This step is unnecessary with sufficient input, but with low input samples, excess primers may be overamplified and contaminate the final library.

To eliminate RNA from downstream reactions and disassociate TGIRT, 3µl 1M NaOH was added to each sample and heated at 95°C for 5 minutes. After cooling to room temperature, 3µl 1M HCl was added to each sample to neutralize the reaction. 24µl 95% EtOH and 24µl Ampure XP beads were added to each sample, flicked to mix, and left to incubate for 10 minutes at room temperature (Fishman & A, 2019). Beads were washed twice with 200µl 80% EtOH and resuspended in 4.2µl H_2O and 4µl supernatant was moved to fresh PCR tubes.

Second-strand synthesis master mixes (SS-MM) were prepared with 1µl ButtRT Buffer, 0.3µl MER1R, 0.3µl TGIRT, 2µl 50% PEG3350, and 0.4µl H_2O. SS-MM were mixed as described earlier. 4µl SS-MM was added to cDNA samples, mixed as described earlier, and assembled reactions were left to incubate on ice for 30 minutes.

While incubating, 1µl 20mM dNTPs was mixed with 10µl 2M NaCl. After 30 minutes, 2µl dNTPs/NaCl mixture was added to TGIRT and placed on the thermal cycler with the following program: 25°C for 1 minute, ramping to 60°C at 1°C/second, 60°C for 30 seconds, then holding at 4°C. Reactions were moved on to ice, and 1µl 0.2% SDS was added to each reaction to disassociate TGIRT. Reactions were incubated 55°C, then moved to room temperature. 30µl Ampure XP beads were added to each reaction, incubated for 5 minutes at room temperature, washed twice, and then eluted in 9µl H_2O.

dsDNA was added to PCR reactions containing 25µl 2x NEBNext Ultra II Q5 Master mix, 2.5µl P7 primer (CAAGCAGAAGACGGCATACGAG), 2.5µl barcoded Ad1 primer(AATGATACGGCGACCACCGAGATCTACAC<Barcode>TCGTCGGCAGCGTCAG ATGTGTAT), and 11µl H_2O. The assembled PCR reaction was subject to the following PCR program: 72°C for 3 minutes, 98°C for 30 seconds, 9-15 cycles of 98°C for 15 seconds and 65°C for 30 seconds, a final extension of 72°C for 2 minutes, and hold at 10°C.

PCR reactions were cleaned with 65µl Ampure XP beads following the standard protocol and resuspended in 10µl 1x Purple Loading Dye. Samples were loaded onto an 8% TBE gel alongside 1µl of TriDye Ultra Low Range DNA ladder mixed with 9µl 1x Purple Loading Dye and run at 180v for 45 minutes. Gels were post-stained with 1x Sybr Gold for 5 minutes, and the smear above 150nt were excised into a 0.5ml tube. The maximum fragment size produced in this protocol should be around ~700nt. For an example gel, please see supplementary table

The gel extraction consists of a "crush and soak" protocol, slightly adapted (Zubradt et al., 2017). 0.5ml tubes had a hole poked in the bottom with a 21-gauge needle and nested inside a 2.0ml tube and centrifuged for 21000g for 3 minutes. If any gel fragments remained in the 0.5ml tube, a second hole was poked and centrifuged again. 600µl 300mM NaCl was added to each tube, and tubes were incubated at 75°C for 15 minutes or 4°C overnight, preferably with agitation or shaking. Supernatant and gel fragments were transferred into a Costar Spin-X Centrifuge Tube Filter with a wide-bore 1000µl pipette tip, or a 1000µl pipette tip with the tip cut off, and spun for 2 minutes at 21000g. Filters were discarded and 600µl isopropanol and 0.7µl GlycoBlue was added to each tube, and left to incubate for at least 15 minutes at room temperature or in -20°C for up to overnight (Li et al., 2020). Samples were spun at 21000g for 30 minutes, washed twice with 80% EtOH, and resuspended in 7-10μl MilliQ H_2O. 2μl was used for analysis on a Tapestation 4200 D1000 tape and quantified using peak quantification centered around 170nt. Samples were sequenced on a NextSeq 500 with at least 8bp dual index reads. Using Drosophila, we sequenced to a depth of at least 20 million paired end reads.

Butt-Seq Data Processing

A snakemake file for analyzing Butt-Seq is available at https://github.com/albertdyu/BuTTSeq , which includes all custom scripts mentioned. Prior to demultiplexing, RunInfo.xml was altered so that Read 2 is not counted as an Indexed read, and samples were demultiplexed using the i5 index. This will output three files: Read 1 corresponds to Read 1, Read 2 corresponds to the UMI, and Read 3 corresponds to Read 2. UMIs were extracted from Read 2 and appended to Read 1 and 3 individually using umi_tools extract with the following command: extract -I READ2_UMI --extract-method=regex --bc-pattern=--read2-in=READ1_OR_3 --stdout=umiextracted_reads/filler.fq.gz --read2-out=OUTPUT.fq.gz (Smith et al., 2017). This will also produce a filler file, which can be deleted. Reads were trimmed using fastp and the following settings: -trim_poly_g --trim_poly_x -F 1 --adapter_sequence AAGATCGGAAGAGC --adapter_sequence_r2 CTGTCTCTTATA (Chen et al., 2018). Reads were subject to 2-pass mapping with STAR to dm6 using the following settings: --alignMatesGapMax 100000 --outSAMstrandField intronMotif --outFilterMismatchNoverLmax 0.05 --outFilterMultimapNmax 1 --outSJfilterReads Unique. Aligned reads were converted to BAM files with Samtools, and deduplicated using umi_tools dedup (Li et al., 2009). Small RNAs and exon 3' ends were computationally removed using SAMtools and a bed file containing small RNAs and exon 3' ends extracted from RefSeq gene annotations, and soft clipping was removed prior to single-nucleotide read conversion using a custom script modified from ngsutils (Breese & Liu, 2013).

Contaminant analysis

For small and non-coding RNA analysis, coordinates for snoRNAs, snRNAs, and scaRNAs were extracted from RefSeq annotation files and used to generate a reference file for featurecounts. Reads mapped to small and non-coding RNAs were quantified using featurecounts, and percentage of reads mapping were reported.

For rRNA analysis, coordinates for rRNA genes were extracted from RefSeq annotation files and used to extract fasta sequences from the dm6 genome assembly. Extracted fasta files were used to build a bowtie2 index, and reads were mapped using bowtie2 with the following settings: --very-fast-local --phred33 --no-mixed --no-discordant --dovetail -I 10 -X 700. Percentage of mapped reads are reported.

Pro-Seq and 3NT-Seq Data Processing

Fastq files were obtained from the SRA using fasterq-dump and aligned to dm6 using STAR with the following settings: --alignMatesGapMax 50000 --outFilterMismatchNoverLmax 0.06 --outFilterMatchNmin 15 --outFilterMultimapNmax 1 --outSJfilterReads Unique. Aligned reads were converted to BAM files with Samtools (Li et al., 2009). Reads were truncated to the first nucleotide of Read 2 using a custom script, get_SNR_bam.py, slightly adapter to fit this pipeline (Nojima et al., 2015).

ChIP-Seq Data Processing and Peak Calling

Fastq files were retrieved from the SRA using fasterq-dump and aligned to dm6 with bwa mem. Peaks were called using MACS2 using the following parameters: --nomodel --extsize 200 -q 0.01.

Butt-Seq Pause Analysis

Reads were truncated to the first nucleotide of Read 2 using a custom script and converted into stranded bedgraph files using Deeptools (Nojima et al., 2016; Ramirez et al., 2014). Bedgraph files were restricted to the first 200nt downstream of each TSS genome-wide, with overlapping genes being merged together.

Pause site analysis

Single-nucleotide peaks were called using the Pause-Detection Algorithm (PDA), with a window size of 100, a minimum intensity of 5, 10,000 bootstraps, and a p-value threshold of 0.00001. (Gajos et al., 2021). Single-nucleotide peaks were used as a reference for quantifying single-nucleotide BAM files using featureCounts, and multiple peaks in a single gene were filtered for the highest peak in R (Liao et al., 2014).

Pausing Index Calculation

Rather than calculating pausing indices using fixed regions, pausing regions were calculated with reference to highest pause peak in each gene. Pause regions were defined as the region from the TSS to the highest pause, and elongation regions were defined as 1000bp downstream of the highest pause. We also calculated pause index by measuring signal from -50 to +200 around the TSS and dividing it by signal across the gene body.

Motif analysis

Single-nucleotide peaks were extended 10nt in either direction with bedtools slop and used as a reference to retrieve fasta sequences from the dm6 reference genome using getfasta (Quinlan, 2014). Motifs were generated from fasta sequences using the R package universalmotif.

mNase-Seq analysis

Fastq files were retrieved from the SRA using fasterq-dump and aligned to dm6 with bwa mem using default settings. BAM files were filtered by insert size using SAMtools. Nucleosome positions were called as previously described, except rather than filtering for the downstream nucleosome, entire alignments were first used for unbiased analysis. Following unbiased analysis, the -1 nucleosome was described as any nucleosome that overlapped an annotated TSS. Bedtools was used to determine nucleosome centers and to calculate the distance to the nearest Butt-Seq pause peak (Quinlan, 2014).

H2Av ChIP-Seq analysis.

Peaks were called using MACS2 using the following parameters: --nomodel --extsize 200 -q 0.01 (Zhang et al., 2008).

Data normalization

Across different tissues and techniques, the molecular composition of each sequencing library can vary dramatically. For example, PRO-Seq contains no contaminating small RNA reads, while 3NT-Seq and Butt-Seq consist of approximately 40% small RNA reads (Supplemental Fig. S1A). Normalization by library depth therefore would be inappropriate. Instead, we normalized data by coverage over regions of interest to control for differences in background using the median of ratios method employed in DESeq2 (Love et al., 2014). For each analysis, bed files describing the features of interest were converted into saf files and used as a reference for counting using featureCounts (Liao et al., 2014). Raw count tables were imported into DESeq2, which we used to produce normalized count tables for correlation analyses and scaling factors. Scaling factors were used to produce normalized bigwig files for data visualization using deepTool's bamCoverage function (Ramirez et al., 2014). For metagene plots, signal over the depicted region were used to generate scaling factors.

RNA-Seq analysis

Fastq files were retrieved from the SRA using fasterq-dump and aligned to dm6 using STAR with the following settings: --alignMatesGapMax 50000 --outFilterMismatchNoverLmax 0.06 --

outFilterMatchNmin 15 --outFilterMultimapNmax 1 --outSJfilterReads Unique. Aligned reads were converted to BAM files with Samtools (Li et al., 2009). Reads were counted using featurecounts using Refseq genes as a reference (Liao et al., 2014). Normalized count files were generated using DESeq2 (Love et al., 2014). For each gene, reads across all timepoints were normalized to the highest timepoint and double-plotted using ggplot2 (Wickham, 2016).

Metagene profiles and gene plots

Mapped reads in each sequencing experiment were used to generate normalization factors with DESeq2 using counts at regions of interest as reference, as described earlier (Love et al., 2014). To simplify visualization, only plus strand reads and genes were used. Coverage plots were scaled to specified regions using deepTools computematrix with a bin size of 1, and the output was used for further processing in R.

In R, outliers defined as the top and bottom 0.1% regions were removed, a pseudo-count of 1 was added to all positions and converted into $\log_2$, from which means and 95% confidence intervals were determined using the bootstrap method with 10,000 repetitions. Means and confidence intervals were plotted using ggplot2(Wickham, 2016). For some figure assembly, Plotgardener was used (Kramer et al., 2022).

Data Availability

Sequencing data has been deposited in the Gene Expression Omnibus (GEO) under the accession code GSE228595. Scripts for data processing and analysis are available at https://github.com/albertdyu/BuTTSeq.

REFERENCES

Abruzzi, K. C., Rodriguez, J., Menet, J. S., Desrochers, J., Zadina, A., Luo, W., Tkachev, S., & Rosbash, M. (2011). Drosophila CLOCK target gene characterization: implications for circadian tissue-specific gene expression. *Genes Dev*, *25*(22), 2374-2386. https://doi.org/10.1101/gad.174110.111
10.1101/gad.178079.111

Adelman, K., & Lis, J. T. (2012). Promoter-proximal pausing of RNA polymerase II: emerging roles in metazoans. *Nat Rev Genet*, *13*(10), 720-731. https://doi.org/10.1038/nrg3293

Begik, O., Diensthuber, G., Liu, H., Delgado-Tejedor, A., Kontur, C., Niazi, A. M., Valen, E., Giraldez, A. J., Beaudoin, J. D., Mattick, J. S., & Novoa, E. M. (2023). Nano3P-seq: transcriptome-wide analysis of gene expression and tail dynamics using end-capture nanopore cDNA sequencing. *Nat Methods*, *20*(1), 75-85. https://doi.org/10.1038/s41592-022-01714-w

Breese, M. R., & Liu, Y. (2013). NGSUtils: a software suite for analyzing and manipulating next-generation sequencing datasets. *Bioinformatics*, *29*(4), 494-496. https://doi.org/10.1093/bioinformatics/bts731

Chen, S., Zhou, Y., Chen, Y., & Gu, J. (2018). fastp: an ultra-fast all-in-one FASTQ preprocessor. *Bioinformatics*, *34*(17), i884-i890. https://doi.org/10.1093/bioinformatics/bty560

Churchman, L. S., & Weissman, J. S. (2012). Native elongating transcript sequencing (NET-seq). *Curr Protoc Mol Biol*, *Chapter 4*, Unit 4 14 11-17. https://doi.org/10.1002/0471142727.mb0414s98

Core, L. J., Waterfall, J. J., & Lis, J. T. (2008). Nascent RNA sequencing reveals widespread pausing and divergent initiation at human promoters. *Science*, *322*(5909), 1845-1848. https://doi.org/10.1126/science.1162228

Dahlberg, O., Shilkova, O., Tang, M., Holmqvist, P. H., & Mannervik, M. (2015). P-TEFb, the super elongation complex and mediator regulate a subset of non-paused genes during early Drosophila embryo development. *PLoS Genet*, *11*(2), e1004971. https://doi.org/10.1371/journal.pgen.1004971

Day, D. S., Zhang, B., Stevens, S. M., Ferrari, F., Larschan, E. N., Park, P. J., & Pu, W. T. (2016). Comprehensive analysis of promoter-proximal RNA polymerase II pausing across mammalian cell types. *Genome Biol*, *17*(1), 120. https://doi.org/10.1186/s13059-016-0984-2

Fishman, A., & A, T. L. (2019). QsRNA-seq: A protocol for generating libraries for high-throughput sequencing of small RNAs. *Bio Protoc*, *9*(5), e3179. https://doi.org/10.21769/BioProtoc.3179

Fong, N., Sheridan, R. M., Ramachandran, S., & Bentley, D. L. (2022). The pausing zone and control of RNA polymerase II elongation by Spt5: Implications for the pause-release model. *Mol Cell*, *82*(19), 3632-3645 e3634. https://doi.org/10.1016/j.molcel.2022.09.001

Gajos, M., Jasnovidova, O., van Bommel, A., Freier, S., Vingron, M., & Mayer, A. (2021). Conserved DNA sequence features underlie pervasive RNA polymerase pausing. *Nucleic Acids Res*, *49*(8), 4402-4420. https://doi.org/10.1093/nar/gkab208

Hardin, P. E. (2005). The circadian timekeeping system of Drosophila. *Curr Biol*, *15*(17), R714-722. https://doi.org/10.1016/j.cub.2005.08.019

He, Q., Johnston, J., & Zeitlinger, J. (2015). ChIP-nexus enables improved detection of in vivo transcription factor binding footprints. *Nat Biotechnol*, *33*(4), 395-401. https://doi.org/10.1038/nbt.3121

Jonkers, I., & Lis, J. T. (2015). Getting up to speed with transcription elongation by RNA polymerase II. *Nat Rev Mol Cell Biol*, *16*(3), 167-177. https://doi.org/10.1038/nrm3953

Judd, J., Wojenski, L. A., Wainman, L. M., Tippens, N. D., Rice, E. J., Dziubek, A., Villafano, G. J., Wissink, E. M., Versluis, P., Bagepalli, L., Shah, S. R., Mahat, D. B., Tome, J. M., Danko, C. G., Lis, J. T., & Core, L. J. (2020). A rapid, sensitive, scalable method for Precision Run-On sequencing (PRO-seq). *bioRxiv*, 2020.2005.2018.102277. https://doi.org/10.1101/2020.05.18.102277

Khodor, Y. L., Menet, J. S., Tolan, M., & Rosbash, M. (2012). Cotranscriptional splicing efficiency differs dramatically between Drosophila and mouse. *RNA*, *18*(12), 2174-2186. https://doi.org/10.1261/rna.034090.112

Kramer, N. E., Davis, E. S., Wenger, C. D., Deoudes, E. M., Parker, S. M., Love, M. I., & Phanstiel, D. H. (2022). Plotgardener: cultivating precise multi-panel figures in R. *Bioinformatics*, *38*(7), 2042-2045. https://doi.org/10.1093/bioinformatics/btac057

Kuintzle, R. C., Chow, E. S., Westby, T. N., Gvakharia, B. O., Giebultowicz, J. M., & Hendrix, D. A. (2017). Circadian deep sequencing reveals stress-response genes that adopt robust rhythmic expression during aging. *Nat Commun*, *8*, 14529. https://doi.org/10.1038/ncomms14529

Li, H., Handsaker, B., Wysoker, A., Fennell, T., Ruan, J., Homer, N., Marth, G., Abecasis, G., Durbin, R., & Genome Project Data Processing, S. (2009). The Sequence Alignment/Map format and SAMtools. *Bioinformatics*, *25*(16), 2078-2079. https://doi.org/10.1093/bioinformatics/btp352

Li, Y., Chen, S., Liu, N., Ma, L., Wang, T., Veedu, R. N., Li, T., Zhang, F., Zhou, H., Cheng, X., & Jing, X. (2020). A systematic investigation of key factors of nucleic acid precipitation toward optimized DNA/RNA isolation. *Biotechniques*, *68*(4), 191-199. https://doi.org/10.2144/btn-2019-0109

Liang, K., Smith, E. R., Aoi, Y., Stoltz, K. L., Katagi, H., Woodfin, A. R., Rendleman, E. J., Marshall, S. A., Murray, D. C., Wang, L., Ozark, P. A., Mishra, R. K., Hashizume, R., Schiltz, G. E., & Shilatifard, A. (2018). Targeting Processive Transcription Elongation via SEC Disruption for MYC-Induced Cancer Therapy. *Cell*, *175*(3), 766-779 e717. https://doi.org/10.1016/j.cell.2018.09.027

Liao, Y., Smyth, G. K., & Shi, W. (2014). featureCounts: an efficient general purpose program for assigning sequence reads to genomic features. *Bioinformatics*, *30*(7), 923-930. https://doi.org/10.1093/bioinformatics/btt656

Love, M. I., Huber, W., & Anders, S. (2014). Moderated estimation of fold change and dispersion for RNA-seq data with DESeq2. *Genome Biol*, *15*(12), 550. https://doi.org/10.1186/s13059-014-0550-8

Mahat, D. B., Kwak, H., Booth, G. T., Jonkers, I. H., Danko, C. G., Patel, R. K., Waters, C. T., Munson, K., Core, L. J., & Lis, J. T. (2016). Base-pair-resolution genome-wide mapping of active RNA polymerases using precision nuclear run-on (PRO-seq). *Nat Protoc*, *11*(8), 1455-1476. https://doi.org/10.1038/nprot.2016.086

Mayer, A., di Iulio, J., Maleri, S., Eser, U., Vierstra, J., Reynolds, A., Sandstrom, R., Stamatoyannopoulos, J. A., & Churchman, L. S. (2015). Native elongating transcript sequencing reveals human transcriptional activity at nucleotide resolution. *Cell*, *161*(3), 541-554. https://doi.org/10.1016/j.cell.2015.03.010

Mayer, A., Landry, H. M., & Churchman, L. S. (2017). Pause & go: from the discovery of RNA polymerase pausing to its functional implications. *Curr Opin Cell Biol*, *46*, 72-80. https://doi.org/10.1016/j.ceb.2017.03.002

Mohr, S., Ghanem, E., Smith, W., Sheeter, D., Qin, Y., King, O., Polioudakis, D., Iyer, V. R., Hunicke-Smith, S., Swamy, S., Kuersten, S., & Lambowitz, A. M. (2013). Thermostable group II intron reverse transcriptase fusion proteins and their use in cDNA synthesis and next-generation RNA sequencing. *RNA*, *19*(7), 958-970. https://doi.org/10.1261/rna.039743.113

Nechaev, S., Fargo, D. C., dos Santos, G., Liu, L., Gao, Y., & Adelman, K. (2010). Global analysis of short RNAs reveals widespread promoter-proximal stalling and arrest of Pol II in Drosophila. *Science*, *327*(5963), 335-338. https://doi.org/10.1126/science.1181421

Nojima, T., Gomes, T., Carmo-Fonseca, M., & Proudfoot, N. J. (2016). Mammalian NET-seq analysis defines nascent RNA profiles and associated RNA processing genome-wide. *Nat Protoc*, *11*(3), 413-428. https://doi.org/10.1038/nprot.2016.012

Nojima, T., Gomes, T., Grosso, A. R. F., Kimura, H., Dye, M. J., Dhir, S., Carmo-Fonseca, M., & Proudfoot, N. J. (2015). Mammalian NET-Seq Reveals Genome-wide Nascent Transcription Coupled to RNA Processing. *Cell*, *161*(3), 526-540. https://doi.org/10.1016/j.cell.2015.03.027

Quinlan, A. R. (2014). BEDTools: The Swiss-Army Tool for Genome Feature Analysis. *Curr Protoc Bioinformatics*, *47*, 11 12 11-34. https://doi.org/10.1002/0471250953.bi1112s47

Ramachandran, S., Ahmad, K., & Henikoff, S. (2017). Transcription and Remodeling Produce Asymmetrically Unwrapped Nucleosomal Intermediates. *Mol Cell*, *68*(6), 1038-1053 e1034. https://doi.org/10.1016/j.molcel.2017.11.015

Ramirez, F., Dundar, F., Diehl, S., Gruning, B. A., & Manke, T. (2014). deepTools: a flexible platform for exploring deep-sequencing data. *Nucleic Acids Res*, *42*(Web Server issue), W187-191. https://doi.org/10.1093/nar/gku365

Rhee, S. S., & Burke, D. H. (2004). Tris(2-carboxyethyl)phosphine stabilization of RNA: comparison with dithiothreitol for use with nucleic acid and thiophosphoryl chemistry. *Anal Biochem*, *325*(1), 137-143. https://doi.org/10.1016/j.ab.2003.10.019

Rodriguez, J., Tang, C. H., Khodor, Y. L., Vodala, S., Menet, J. S., & Rosbash, M. (2013). Nascent-Seq analysis of Drosophila cycling gene expression. *Proc Natl Acad Sci U S A*, *110*(4), E275-284. https://doi.org/10.1073/pnas.1219969110

Schlackow, M., Nojima, T., Gomes, T., Dhir, A., Carmo-Fonseca, M., & Proudfoot, N. J. (2017). Distinctive Patterns of Transcription and RNA Processing for Human lincRNAs. *Mol Cell*, *65*(1), 25-38. https://doi.org/10.1016/j.molcel.2016.11.029

Smith, T., Heger, A., & Sudbery, I. (2017). UMI-tools: modeling sequencing errors in Unique Molecular Identifiers to improve quantification accuracy. *Genome Res*, *27*(3), 491-499. https://doi.org/10.1101/gr.209601.116

So, W. V., & Rosbash, M. (1997). Post-transcriptional regulation contributes to Drosophila clock gene mRNA cycling. *EMBO J*, *16*(23), 7146-7155. https://doi.org/10.1093/emboj/16.23.7146

Sousa-Luis, R., Dujardin, G., Zukher, I., Kimura, H., Weldon, C., Carmo-Fonseca, M., Proudfoot, N. J., & Nojima, T. (2021). POINT technology illuminates the processing of polymerase-associated intact nascent transcripts. *Mol Cell*, *81*(9), 1935-1950 e1936. https://doi.org/10.1016/j.molcel.2021.02.034

Taylor, P., & Hardin, P. E. (2008). Rhythmic E-box binding by CLK-CYC controls daily cycles in per and tim

transcription and chromatin modifications. *Mol Cell Biol*, *28*(14), 4642-4652. https://doi.org/10.1128/MCB.01612-07
Weber, C. M., Ramachandran, S., & Henikoff, S. (2014). Nucleosomes are context-specific, H2A.Z-modulated barriers to RNA polymerase. *Mol Cell*, *53*(5), 819-830. https://doi.org/10.1016/j.molcel.2014.02.014
Wickham, H. (2016). *Ggplot2 : elegant graphics for data analysis*. Springer Science+Business Media, LLC.
Wissink, E. M., Vihervaara, A., Tippens, N. D., & Lis, J. T. (2019). Nascent RNA analyses: tracking transcription and its regulation. *Nat Rev Genet*, *20*(12), 705-723. https://doi.org/10.1038/s41576-019-0159-6
Wu, D. C., & Lambowitz, A. M. (2017). Facile single-stranded DNA sequencing of human plasma DNA via thermostable group II intron reverse transcriptase template switching. *Sci Rep*, *7*(1), 8421. https://doi.org/10.1038/s41598-017-09064-w
Wuarin, J., & Schibler, U. (1994). Physical isolation of nascent RNA chains transcribed by RNA polymerase II: evidence for cotranscriptional splicing. *Mol Cell Biol*, *14*(11), 7219-7225. https://doi.org/10.1128/mcb.14.11.7219-7225.1994
Xu, H., Nottingham, R. M., & Lambowitz, A. M. (2021). TGIRT-seq Protocol for the Comprehensive Profiling of Coding and Non-coding RNA Biotypes in Cellular, Extracellular Vesicle, and Plasma RNAs. *Bio Protoc*, *11*(23), e4239. https://doi.org/10.21769/BioProtoc.4239
Yao, J., Wu, D. C., Nottingham, R. M., & Lambowitz, A. M. (2020). Identification of protein-protected mRNA fragments and structured excised intron RNAs in human plasma by TGIRT-seq peak calling. *Elife*, *9*. https://doi.org/10.7554/eLife.60743
Zhang, Y., Liu, T., Meyer, C. A., Eeckhoute, J., Johnson, D. S., Bernstein, B. E., Nusbaum, C., Myers, R. M., Brown, M., Li, W., & Liu, X. S. (2008). Model-based analysis of ChIP-Seq (MACS). *Genome Biol*, *9*(9), R137. https://doi.org/10.1186/gb-2008-9-9-r137
Zubradt, M., Gupta, P., Persad, S., Lambowitz, A. M., Weissman, J. S., & Rouskin, S. (2017). DMS-MaPseq for genome-wide or targeted RNA structure probing in vivo. *Nat Methods*, *14*(1), 75-82. https://doi.org/10.1038/nmeth.4057

FIGURES AND FIGURE LEGENDS

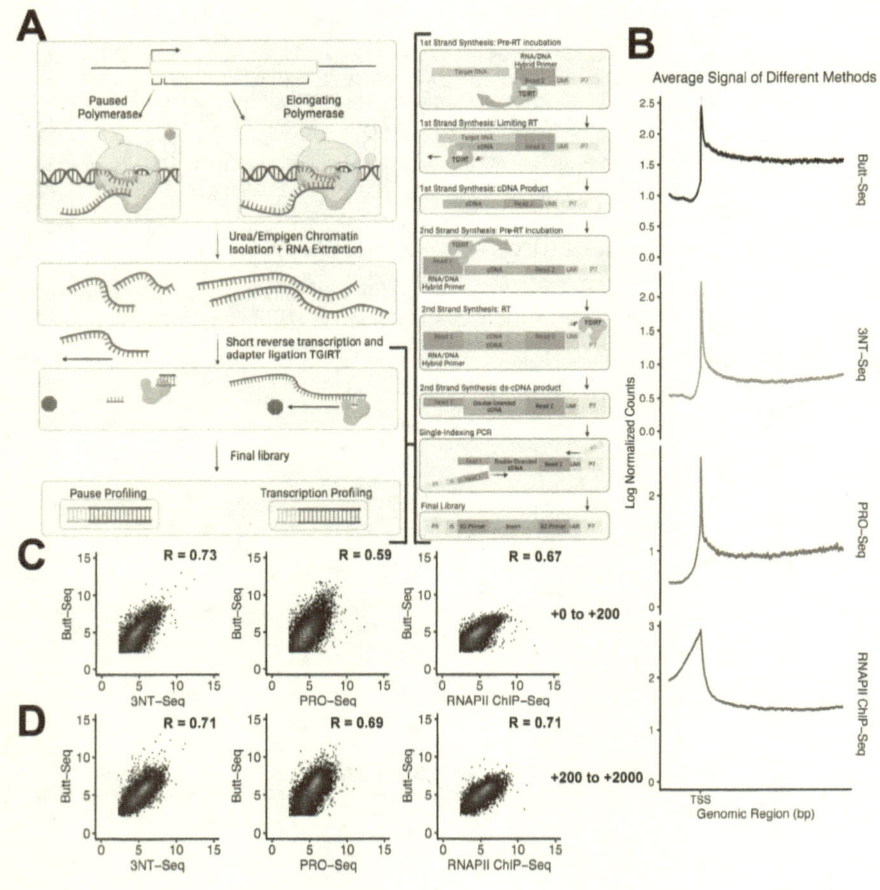

Figure 1. Butt-Seq measures transcription and is comparable to other transcription analysis methods.

(A) Butt-Seq-method overview. Figure was created with Biorender.

(B) Scaled metagene plots of signal distribution in plus strand genes over 5kb in length (N=6284) across Butt-Seq, 3NT-Seq, PRO-Seq, and RNAPII ChIP-Seq. On the X axis, the transcription start site (TSS) is marked and plot extends 1kb into the gene body and 200bp upstream. The Y axis represents the log2-transformed normalized signal in each method. The shaded area corresponds to the 95% confidence interval.

(C) Log-log plot of normalized counts from Butt-Seq compared to 3NT-Seq, PRO-Seq, and RNAPII ChIP-Seq genome-wide(N=10744). Signal was quantified from the region 200nt downstream of the TSS genome-wide. The Y-axis represents the log2- transformed Butt-Seq counts, while the X-axis represents the log2-transformed 3NT-Seq(Left), PRO-Seq(Middle), and RNAPII ChIP-Seq(Right) counts. Correlations were calculated using Spearman's rank correlation coefficient.

(D) Log-log plot of normalized counts from Butt-Seq compared to 3NT-Seq, PRO-Seq, and RNAPII ChIP-Seq genome-wide(N=. Signal was quantified from the region +200nt to +2000nt downstream of the TSS. The Y-axis represents the log2-transformed Butt-Seq counts, while the X-axis represents the log2-transformed 3NT- Seq(Left), PRO-Seq(Middle), and RNAPII ChIP-Seq(Right) counts. Correlations were calculated using Spearman's rank correlation coefficient.

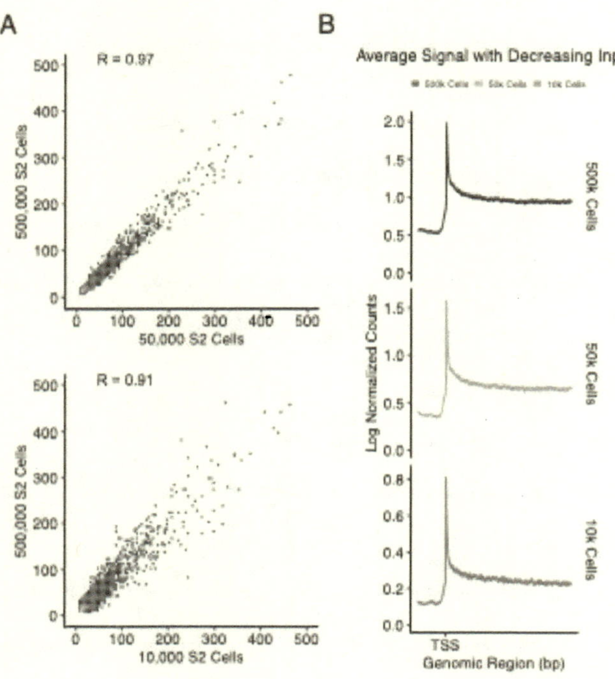

Figure 2. Butt-Seq signal is reproducible down to 10,000 cells.

(A) Comparison of signal from Butt-Seq data generated from 500,000, 50,000, and 10,000 cells. Signal was quantified from 200nt downstream of the TSS genome-wide. The Y-axis represents the log2-transformed counts from 500,000 cells, while the X-axis represents the log2-transformed counts from 50,000 (Top) and 10,000 (Bottom) cells.

(B) Metagene plots of signal distribution in plus strand genes over 5kb in length (N=6284) from 500,000, 50,000, and 10,000 cells. On the X axis, the transcription start site (TSS) is marked and plot extends 1kb into the gene body and 200bp upstream. The Y axis represents the log2-transformed normalized signal in each method. Data was normalized to the depicted region The shaded area corresponds to the 95% confidence interval.

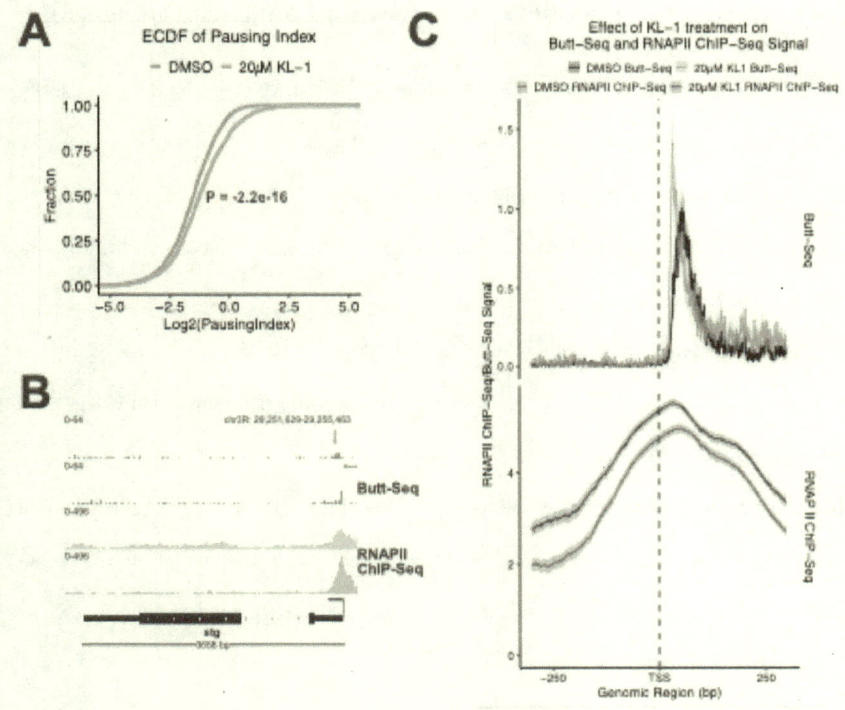
A
ECDF of Pausing Index
DMSO
20μM KL-1
P = -2.2e-16
Fraction
Log2(PausingIndex)
B
Butt-Seq
RNAPII
ChIP-Seq
C
Effect of KL-1 treatment on
Butt-Seq and RNAPII ChIP-Seq Signal
Butt-Seq
RNAP II ChIP-Seq
Genomic Region (bp)

Figure 3. Butt-Seq recapitulates pausing dynamics seen in RNAPII ChIP-Seq upon KL-1 treatment.

(A) ECDF of pausing index in Butt-Seq in S2 cells treated with DMSO or 20μM KL-1. Pausing region is defined as the region from the TSS to the highest pause site determined by pause detection algorithm (PDA), and gene body region is defined as 1000nt downstream of each pause site.The Y-axis depicts the cumulative fraction of genes, while the X-axis contains the log2-transformed pausing index.

(B) Representative gene demonstrating the effect of 20μM KL-1 treatment on signal distribution in Butt-Seq and RNAPII ChIP-Seq. Green arrow: Untreated pause site. Purple arrow: KL-1 induced pause site.

(C) Metagene plots of log2-normalized Butt-Seq and RNAPII ChIP-Seq counts, centered around RNAPII ChIP-Seq peaks called from DMSO-treated S2 cells that overlap with Butt-Seq single-nucleotide pause peaks. Only plus strand genes are depicted (N=219). Shade region represents the 95% confidence interval.

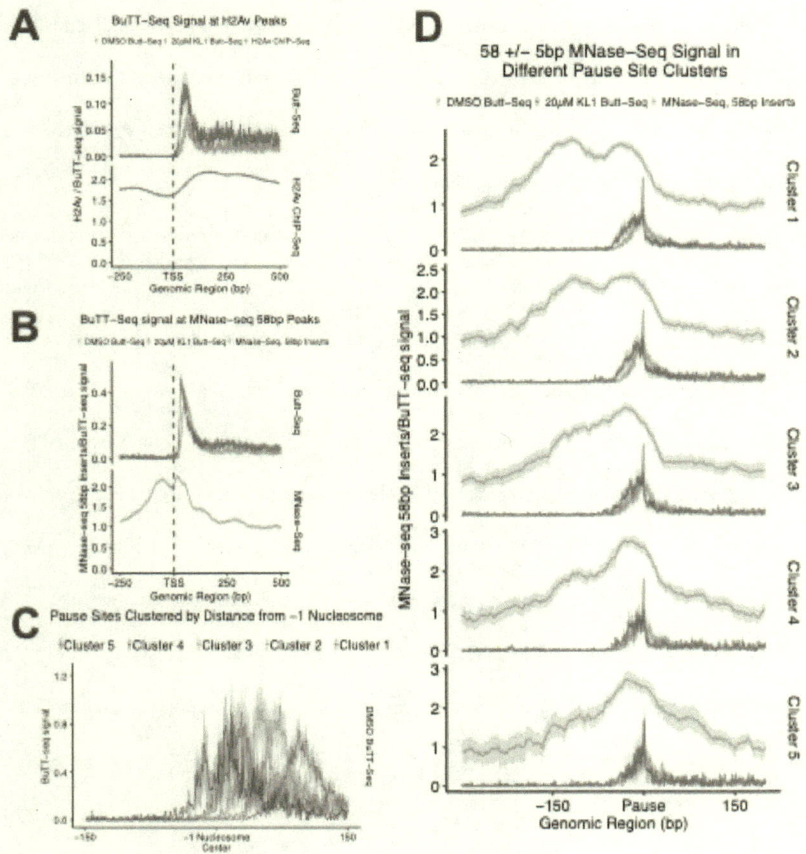
A
BuTT-Seq Signal at H2Av Peaks
H2Av / BuTT-seq signal
Butt-Seq
H2Av ChIP-Seq
Genomic Region (bp)
B
BuTT-Seq signal at MNase-seq 58bp Peaks
MNase-seq 58bp Inserts/BuTT-seq signal
MNase-Seq
Genomic Region (bp)
C
Pause Sites Clustered by Distance from -1 Nucleosome
Cluster 5
Cluster 4
Cluster 3
Cluster 2
Cluster 1
BuTT-seq signal
DMSO BuTT-Seq
-1 Nucleosome Center
Genomic Region (bp)
D
58 +/- 5bp MNase-Seq Signal in Different Pause Site Clusters
DMSO Butt-Seq
20µM KL1 Butt-Seq
MNase-Seq, 58bp Inserts
MNase-seq 58bp Inserts/BuTT-seq signal
Cluster 1
Cluster 2
Cluster 3
Cluster 4
Cluster 5
-150
Pause
150
Genomic Region (bp)

Figure 4. Pausing as assayed by Butt-Seq is correlated with nucleosomal dynamics.

(A) Metagene plots of log2-transformed Butt-Seq counts compared to log2-normalized MNase-seq counts, restricted to 58bp +/- 5nt fragments from MNase-seq. Plotted genes were derived from MNase-seq peaks that overlap with annotated TSS; plus-strand genes are shown (N=831). Shaded area corresponds to 95% confidence interval.

(B) Metagene plot of log2-transformed H2Av ChIP-Seq counts compared to log2-transformed Butt-Seq counts from S2 cells treated with DMSO or 20μM KL-1. Plotted genes were derived from H2Av ChIP-seq peaks that overlap with annotated TSS; plus-strand genes are shown (N=1531). Shaded area corresponds to 95% confidence interval.

(C) Clustering of pause peaks based on distance from the -1 nucleosome center. Depicted are plus strand genes. Cluster 1 contains pauses 80-120bp downstream (N=140), Cluster 2 contains pauses 60-79bp downstream (N=95), Cluster 3 40-59bp (N=63), Cluster 4 20-39bp (N=45), and Cluster 5 0-19bp. (N=35). The shaded area corresponds to the 95% confidence interval.

(D) Metagene plot of log2-normalized 58bp +/- 5bp MNase-Seq counts against log2-normalized KL-1 and DMSO treated Butt-Seq counts across 5 clusters. Shaded area corresponds to 95% confidence interval.

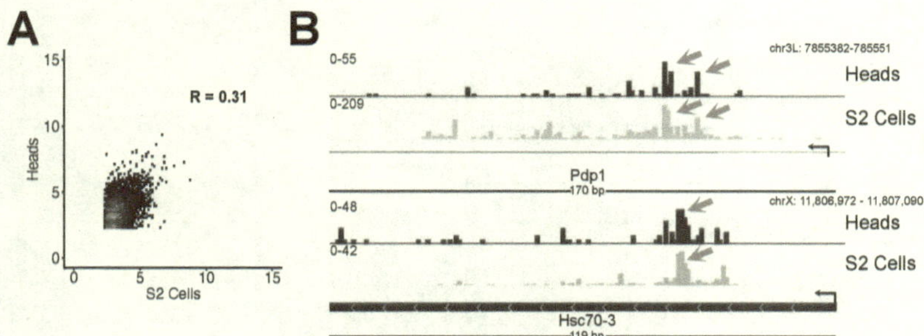

Figure 5. Despite low correlation in gene expression, S2 cells and heads share similar pausing features in co-expressed genes.

(A) Comparison of counts from Butt-Seq data generated from S2 cells or heads. Signal was quantified from 200nt downstream of the TSS genome-wide. The Y-axis represents the log2-transformed counts from heads, while the X-axis represents the log2-transformed counts from S2 cells.

(B) Representative genome browser view of genes exhibiting similar pause sites in heads and S2 cells. Green arrow: Representative shared pause sites.

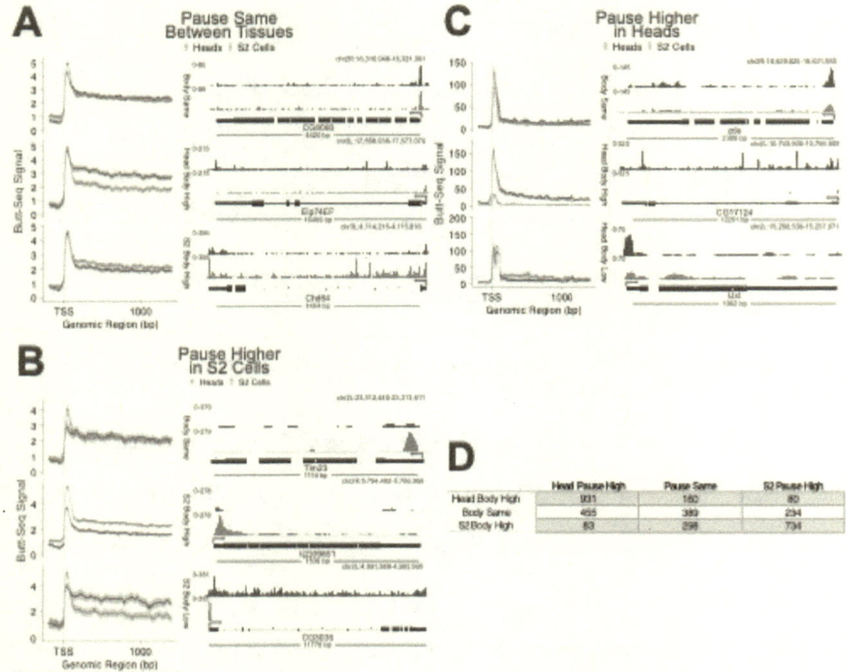

	Head Pause High	Pause Same	S2 Pause High
Head Body High	931	160	80
Body Same	455	389	234
S2 Body High	83	298	734

Figure 6. Differential analysis of Butt-Seq in heads and S2 cells reveals a diverse range of transcriptional programs. Metagene analysis (left) and representative genes (right) reflecting different combinations of pause region and gene body signal between S2 cells and heads.

(A) Pausing is the same between heads and S2 cells.

(B) Pausing is higher in S2 cells.

(C) Pausing is higher in heads.

(D) Total number of genes occupying each pause/gene body combination.

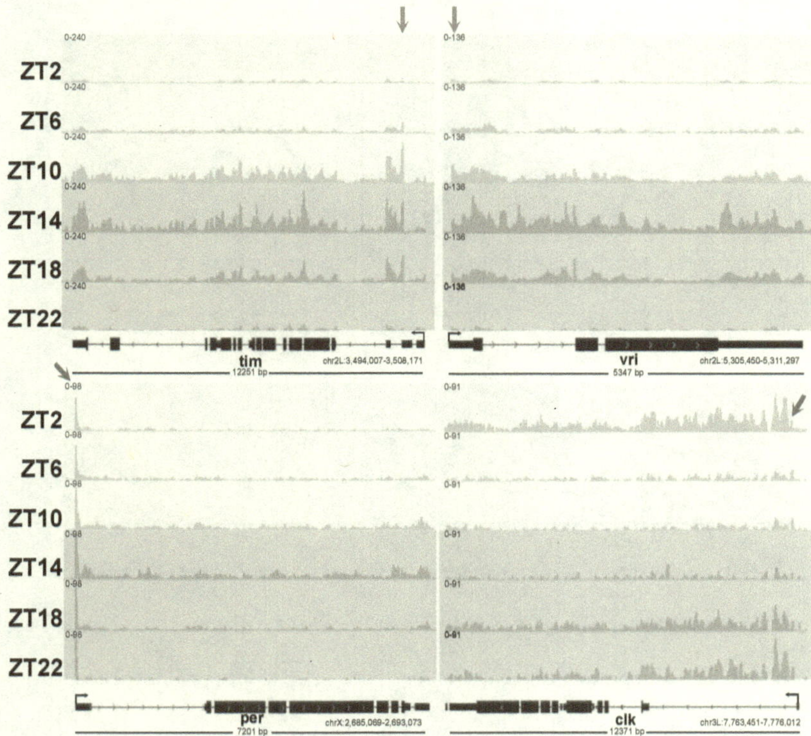

Figure 7. Butt-Seq exhibits transcriptional cycling of core circadian genes. Genome browser view of six timepoints of core circadian genes in Butt-Seq. Green Arrow: Cycling pause. Purple arrow: Constant pause.

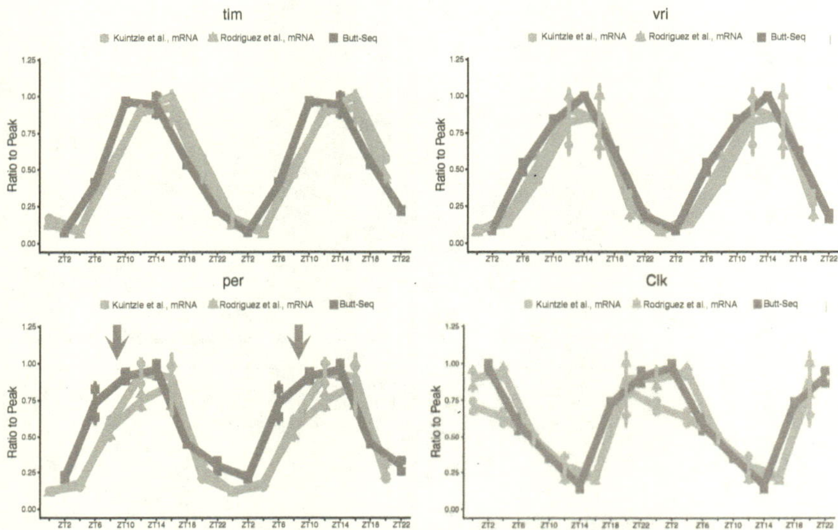

Figure 8. Butt-Seq recapitulates known transcriptional features of the Circadian clock. Butt-Seq double-plotted against RNA-Seq data from Rodriguez et al. (2013) and Kuintzle et al. (2017) at core circadian genes. Each timepoint was normalized to the peak timepoint in respective genes. Green arrow: "Hump" of transcription in per gene.

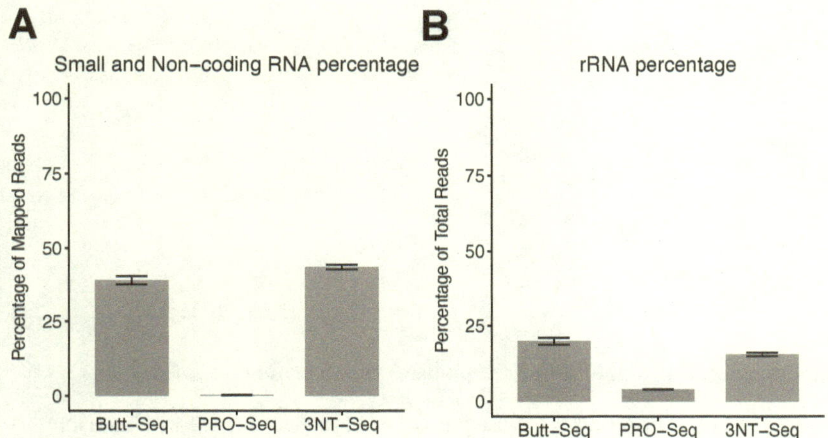

Supplementary Figure 1. Contaminant measures in different techniques.

(A) Percentage of mapped reads that map to snoRNAs, snRNAs, and scaRNAs.

(B) Percentage of total reads that map to a custom genome annotation containing only rRNA.

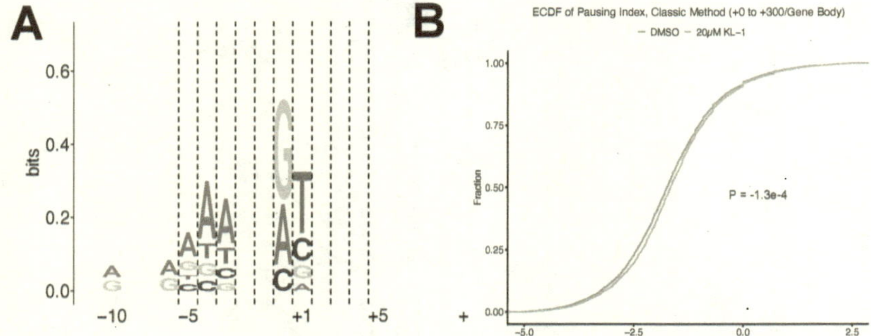

Supplementary Figure 2. Butt-Seq recapitulates known features of pausing.

(A) Motif identified from Butt-Seq pauses located within 200nt downstream of the TSS identified by PDA.

(B) ECDF of pausing index in Butt-Seq in S2 cells treated with DMSO or 20μM KL-1. Pausing index here is defined as -50 to +200 around the TSS divided by signal across the gene body.

CHAPTER 4

Development and Application of VibeCheck in Circadian Transcriptomics

Albert D. Yu[1], Michael Rosbash[1]*

1 Department of Biology, Howard Hughes Medical Institute and National Center for Behavioral Genomics, Brandeis University, Waltham, MA 02453, USA

INTRODUCTION

Circadian biology and the identification of cycling molecules has been faced with unusually high sampling requirements and has long had to balance collecting enough experimental timepoints to determine rhythmicity against cost and effort. Historically, 4–6-hour resolution was considered sufficient, and rhythmicity could be assessed qualitatively – by plotting for example -- on low-throughput experiments (Hughes et al., 2017). High throughput technology renders such qualitative assessment unfeasible, and many computational approaches have been developed to identify rhythmic oscillations in large datasets and distinguish them from oscillation patterns that may have arisen by chance (Agostinelli et al., 2016; Hughes et al., 2010; Hutchison et al., 2018; Thaben & Westermark, 2014; Wu et al., 2016).

Commensurate with the proliferation of high-throughput technology came the realization that 4-hour resolution was insufficient for identifying rhythmicity. Analyses of down-sampled and simulated data suggested that a minimum 2-hour sampling resolution was necessary for the statistical identification of rhythms (Hughes et al., 2017; Hughes et al., 2009); however, this realization was not accompanied by wide-spread adoption of high-resolution sampling schemes. Such reluctance is unsurprising: doubling the number of samples can more than double the labor and cost involved, while also introducing increased technical variation.

The impact of such reluctance varies depending on the nature of the study. For functional hypothesis generation, accompanied by independent validation, it's largely inconsequential. However, many circadian studies draw major conclusions solely based on differential rhythmicity. With underpowered experiments, the extent of differential rhythmicity tends to be exaggerated

(Pelikan et al., 2022).

This story begins with the presence of an intrinsic molecular clock – a set of transcription factors whose rhythmic expression governs all other rhythms - conserved across multiple domains of life (Andreani et al., 2015; Patke et al., 2020). The existence of such "core clock genes" suggested that these transcription factors represented the tip of the iceberg of a much broader program of intrinsically oscillating genes. However, early microarray experiments were marked by a surprising absence of overlap in rhythmic transcripts. This discrepancy was later partially resolved through the application of more expansive statistical examination, which expanded the extent of the known intrinsic clock but likely did not identify it in its entirety (Keegan et al., 2007). A corollary of an intrinsic clock is that there is also like to be an extrinsic clock – rhythmic genes that are mediated by environmental factors, such as light and feeding. Such genes may also vary from lab to lab. The extent of the intrinsic and the extrinsic clock is an outstanding question in the field.

Since the introduction of high-throughput sequencing, ever-growing numbers of "around-the-clock" studies are being performed. Chief among these are studies examining mouse liver, which has emerged as an archetypal circadian tissue owing to its homogeneity and facile collection. We sought to identify intrinsically oscillating genes by reanalyzing high-throughput mouse liver datasets - 23 in all - and finding common oscillations between these datasets. Re-analysis of mouse liver datasets reiterates the importance of appropriate experimental design – in 4 hour resolution datasets with 2 replicates, a median of approximately 800 genes are identified as rhythmic, while in 2 hour resolution datasets, between 3000 to 5000 genes are identified as rhythmic. Graphing rhythmic genes in high resolution datasets, however, reveals another problem – the potential existence of false positives. Many statistically significant cyclers in high resolution datasets do not present convincing visual evidence of cycling making their existence questionable.

We obtained a broad estimate of intrinsic cyclers by identifying genes that are commonly cycling in most datasets, totaling approximately 2000 genes. We reasoned that these genes are likely cycling in all datasets or are at least bona fide cycling transcripts (intrinsic cyclers) but aren't called as cycling due to deficiencies in experimental design and execution in some datasets. Nonetheless, we leveraged these cyclers by training a neural network to then identify transcriptional oscillations in underpowered data, for example 4 hour time point data, which we call VibeCheck. While VibeCheck performs similarly to existing approaches on synthetic data, it exhibits superior performance whenever there is substantial noise - suggesting that VibeCheck may be more robust in the face of experimental error or underpowered data. The latter is often the case as labs tend to collect four hour time points, 6/24 hrs, for obvious practical reasons.

We used VibeCheck to identify an intrinsic clock in *Drosophila* heads, where we observed a potential oscillating transcriptional program mediated by novel transcription factors, namely, *Sp1* and *brk*. Examining these intrinsic cyclers against nascent RNA identified from Butt-Seq data indicated that transcriptional cycling was apparent in approximately 70% of these genes. We then used VibeCheck to identify common and unique cyclers from single cell data in *Drosophila* clock neurons, where we found many cyclers in common across all clusters and identified potential transcription factors mediating unique oscillations in some clusters.

VibeCheck is not a tool to generate a definitive list of cyclers. Rather, it is a tool to pull as many genes as possible with evidence of cycling from a transcriptomic dataset, with the intent for the end-user to adjust thresholds as necessary to suit their intended follow-up experiments; it is not intended to generate a final dataset on its own. Moreover, our analyses revealed a common theme: the need to validate statistical observations through graphing and visualization. Thus, we present VibeCheck as a tool to help refine and generate hypotheses and demonstrate a few potential use cases for VibeCheck.

RESULTS

VibeCheck is a neural network trained on experimental circadian transcriptomic data with the aim of identifying rhythmic transcripts in the most common source of circadian data, namely noisy and under sampled data. We leveraged 23 circadian transcriptomic datasets from mouse liver – representing over a decade of research from investigators around the world - to identify genes that are consistently cycling in a most datasets. These oscillating genes should exhibit rhythmic expression independent of most external environmental factors. We trained VibeCheck to identify these genes as rhythmic in all 23 datasets, thus in principle enabling it to identify rhythmicity across a broad range of experimental variation.

Identifying a set of intrinsic cyclers

To train VibeCheck, we needed to identify a set of consistently oscillating genes, including ones that may have been overlooked by existing algorithms.

We first examined the degree of overlap between the 5 lowest resolution and the 5 highest resolution datasets using JTK Cycle (Hughes et al., 2010). Unsurprisingly, the number of overlapping rhythmic genes in low resolution datasets is quite low – just 83 (Fig 1A). In high resolution datasets, however, the number of commonly cycling genes is considerably higher, at 536 (Fig 1B). This recapitulates previous findings, that the low number of common cyclers is probably related to sampling resolution.

However, this likely does not represent the true breadth of intrinsic cyclers, so we aimed to define a set of cyclers common to most datasets. In order to do so, we needed to first determine the number of datasets to intersect that would give us a high confidence group of cyclers.

A previous study found that algorithms used to detect cycling were prone to both false positives and false negatives at low sampling resolutions (Ness-Cohn et al., 2020). However, this paper did not address the possibility of false positives in high resolution data. Indeed, our plotting data indicated that that some significantly cycling genes were qualitatively unconvincing even from high resolution data (Fig 1C). We therefore simulated finding genes common to as few as 2 to as many as 23 datasets using false positive, false negative, and true positive ratios previously reported in low resolution data in order to maximize our estimation of true positive cyclers. In other words, we wanted to determine how many datasets a gene must appear in for us to call it as consistently cycling.

When simulating intersection using ratios reported for the very common algorithm JTK Cycle, we found that false positives disappear after intersecting 9 datasets, but false negatives also dominate at that point as well (Fig 1D, left). Changes in specificity and sensitivity appeared to observe a logarithmic function, and the approximate midpoint for appearance of false negatives and disappearance for false positives appeared to coincide at 5 datasets. Therefore, we elected to define genes that appear in at least 5 datasets as intrinsic cyclers.

We also decided to include the algorithm RAIN to help determine intrinsically cycling genes (Thaben & Westermark, 2014). Unlike JTK Cycle, RAIN does not require symmetric waveforms, and is thereby capable of detecting rhythms potentially invisible to JTK Cycle. RAIN is also reported to have a significantly higher false positive rate [REF]; indeed, when we simulated intersecting data using false discovery ratios reported for RAIN, we had to intersect 14 datasets to minimize the number of false positives (Fig 1D, right). We therefore called genes that were significantly cycling by RAIN in at least 14 datasets as additional intrinsic cyclers.

When intersecting JTK cycling genes, found in at least 7 datasets, with RAIN cycling genes, found in at least 14 datasets, there were 2044 genes; 1306 were in common between the two methods, and 528 were exclusive to JTK and 210 were exclusive to RAIN Fig 2A). We consider 2/3 in common between the two methods very good correspondence. When plotting a subset of the exclusive genes, they appear to largely be low amplitude cyclers (Fig 2B and 2C). Nonetheless, they appear to have some evidence of cycling with similar phases and amplitudes across datasets, so we used these 2044 intrinsically cycling mouse liver genes for training.

Developing VibeCheck Framework and Architecture

Previous work reports that neural networks outperform other machine learning methods for classifying circadian transcriptomic data as periodic or aperiodic; therefore, we focused on developing a neural network framework to also identify oscillating transcripts (Agostinelli et al., 2016). This previous work used a deep neural network (DNN); however, in our preliminary trials, we found that a long short-term memory network (LSTM) based architecture outperformed DNNs in predicting rhythmicity.

Initially, we performed hyperparameter tuning with separate goals for precision and recall, with the intent to create two separate models for stringent and relaxed parameters for rhythmicity. However, we found that changes in the two parameters tended to coincide, so we focused on optimizing for loss instead. Most hyperparameters had little effect on the model's performance, with two exceptions: A relu activation function for the input LSTM layer significantly reduced overfitting, while the addition of an attention layer improved recall.

We also found that emphasizing the cyclical nature of the data through circular encoding by converting each datapoint to a 2D array with their sine and cosine transformations improved performance of the model as well.

Altogether, the model features an LSTM layer that passes sequences to a global attention layer, followed by two dense layers. The final dense layer is a single-node layer with a sigmoid activation function for binary classification - periodic or aperiodic. VibeCheck outputs a list of genes classified as periodic, along with a "Prediction Value" describing the model's confidence in its classification.

VibeCheck is more resistant to noise than existing approaches

We compared VibeCheck's performance to JTK_Cycle on synthetic 6-timepoint, 2-replicate data generated by CircaInSilico and plotted the receiver operating characteristic (ROC) curve, using ascending P-value for JTK_Cycle and descending Prediction Value for VibeCheck (Hughes et al., 2017).

On a standard output, the performance of both VibeCheck and JTK_Cycle were nearly identical, both achieving an area under curve (AUC) of 0.90 (Fig 3, Top). However, we expect VibeCheck to perform better on noisy data, such as that from underpowered data with experimental error introduced. Thus, we randomly jittered the data by anywhere between 5% and 30% to represent a modest amount of noise, and between 10% to 50% to represent a large amount of noise. With a modest amount of noise, VibeCheck slightly outperforms JTK_Cycle, with an AUC of 0.84 compared to 0.82, respectively (Fig 3, Middle). With a large amount of noise, VibeCheck's performance exhibits remarkable resilience with an AUC of 0.81, compared to 0.68 from JTK_Cycle (Fig 3, Bottom).

Based on these performance metrics, we conclude that VibeCheck potentially outperforms JTK_Cycle at identifying oscillations in noisy data. Thus, on high quality RNA-Seq data, we would anticipate the two approaches to provide similar results – but on data with greater experimental error or sequenced to insufficient depth – a common feature in real world data, VibeCheck may outperform JTK_Cycle.

VibeCheck uncovers intrinsic cyclers in Drosophila heads

The challenge of reproducibility has been a consistent concern in the field of circadian transcriptomics. In our reanalysis of 10 circadian RNA-seq fly head datasets, we discovered that a mere 132 genes were rhythmic with an unadjusted JTK Cycle P-value < 0.01 in only 5 of these 10 data sets. However, with the implementation of VibeCheck, we identified 511 genes, almost 4 times as many, that were commonly rhythmic between at least 5 datasets with a prediction value of over 0.5. These 511 genes included 131 of the 132 commonly rhythmic genes previously identified by JTK Cycle (Fig 4A). When we plotted genes identified as rhythmic by VibeCheck but not JTK Cycle, we found that they qualitatively displayed similar phases and amplitudes across all datasets (6 representative datasets shown for 50 representative genes in Fig 4B). The same trend was observed in the 131 genes as well.

To further explore the methodology, we adjusted our approach to identify what we term as "extrinsic genes," or genes that cycle in only one dataset, potentially due to contribution from different environmental factors or idiosyncratic features that do not replicate across datasets. We altered the thresholds to identify high confidence extrinsic cyclers, setting a Prediction Value threshold of 0.8 for single datasets, and a Prediction Value threshold of 0.1 in at least 4 datasets for the rest. The reduced prediction threshold for intrinsic cycling potentially increases the number of false positives, but it also helps eliminate false negatives, thus improving our confidence in the identified extrinsic cyclers.

During the evaluation of putative extrinsic cyclers, we noted a considerable amount of noise surrounding these cycling genes, and that they were largely lowly expressed in other datasets (Fig 4C). This raises the possibility that at least some extrinsic circadian programs are all-or-nothing – that is to say, if a gene is expressed, it will be expressed rhythmically; however, we could not identify evidence of any common transcriptional programs driving putative extrinsically cycling genes – save for some motifs involved in chromatin architecture, such as M1BP, Beaf-32, and trl (data not shown). The other, perhaps more likely possibility is that the most rhythmically expressed genes are intrinsic, and many extrinsic cyclers might be attributed to experimental error.

VibeCheck suggests the majority of cycling genes are transcriptionally driven

If most circadian genes are indeed intrinsically driven, a potential conclusion may be that their oscillation originates from a shared molecular mechanism, such as transcription. However, the question of what percentage of transcripts oscillate at a transcriptional level has seen varying responses in the past decade, with estimates ranging from 25% to 70% (Atger et al., 2015; Koike et al., 2012; Rodriguez et al., 2013). By utilizing VibeCheck to examine rhythmicity in Bulk Analysis of Nascent Transcript Termini sequencing (Butt-Seq) data, collected from six timepoints (every 4 hours) around the clock, we discovered rhythmicity in 986 transcripts with a Prediction Value threshold of 0.5. 342 of these overlap with the 511 intrinsically cycling genes defined earlier (Fig 5A) (Yu & Rosbash, 2023).

Based on this extent of overlap, we would estimate that at least 67% of oscillating genes are transcriptionally driven - approximately in line with the most recent study to address this question, which is incidentally the most highly powered study as well (Atger et al., 2015). Plotting some of the 644 other Butt-Seq cycling transcripts suggests that ratio largely holds true, and that 511 is likely a very conservative estimate of intrinsically cycling genes (Fig 5B). Altogether, we estimate that approximately 70% of oscillating transcripts are oscillating transcriptionally.

SP1/BRK is a putative transcription complex regulating periodic expression in glia

Though the master transcription factor CLK directly regulates a wide array of genes, it is unlikely to directly account for many, likely most of these intrinsically cycling genes (Abruzzi et al., 2011). To find other transcription factors that may be involved in driving oscillating transcription, we took the intrinsic cyclers and looked for adjacent peaks from CantonS head ATAC-Seq data to identify regulatory regions associated with those genes. We then performed motif analysis on these regions using the MEME suite and Homer (Bailey et al., 2015; Heinz et al., 2010).

As expected, E-boxes were identified by Homer in 49/298 regions - likely representing direct CLK targets (Fig 6A). The top hit identified by MEME, however, was a motif that most closely resembled the Sp1 binding site (Fig 6B). Sp1 has been previously implicated in circadian transcription in mammals through an interaction with Nr1d1 (Mendez-Ferrer et al., 2008); however, its role in Drosophila circadian transcription has not been characterized. Although Sp1 itself does not appear to cycle, one of its binding partners – brk– exhibits modest qualitative evidence of cycling in the majority of datasets (3 representative mRNA-Seq and Butt-Seq plotted in Fig 6C) (Shokri et al., 2019). Regulation of these TFs could of course be post-transcriptional.

We sought to identify other transcripts potentially regulated by SP1/BRK by inverting our previous approach – we subsetted all ATAC-Seq peaks containing an Sp1 motif, then looked for peaks that exhibited differential ATAC-Seq signal between CantonS and ClkJrk – a CLK mutant line that's completely arrhythmic. We hypothesize that because CLK is upstream of all other transcriptional oscillations, any downstream changes in regulatory networks may be reflected through ATAC-Seq in ClkJrk (ATAC-seq experiments conducted by Pranav Ojha). We focused on ATAC-Seq peaks that decreased in ClkJrk, indicative of a loss of a regulatory region (Fig 6D.We then compared differences between ZT2 and ZT14 in CantonS and ClkJrk in nascent RNA sequenced using Butt-seq (Unpublished data).

We found that many putative Sp1 targets that are upregulated at ZT14 in CantonS, but largely exhibited no significant difference between ZT2 and ZT14 in ClkJrk (Fig 6E). This includes brk itself, 6 previously identified intrinsic cyclers, and 36 other genes.

Although we did not recover the brk motif itself from ATAC-Seq, this may be because loss of BRK does not induce chromatin compaction, while loss of SP1 does. However, BRK may nevertheless occlude Tn5 transposition in a more subtle fashion – AKA a transcription factor footprint. We thus compared footprints between ATAC-Seq obtained from CantonS and ClkJrk heads using transcription factor Occupancy prediction By Invesitgation of ATAC-Seq Signal (TOBIAS), where we observed a significant increase in footprints at brk motifs in CantonS – implying the loss of brk binding in ClkJrk (Fig 6F) (Bentsen et al., 2020).

To determine the tissues in which this transcriptional program might be active, we examined single-cell transcriptomic data from heads. Intriguingly, Sp1 and brk were only co-expressed in cells also expressing alrm - a marker gene for astrocyte-like glial cells that are known to be highly rhythmic (Fig 7A, circled in red) (Li et al., 2022). When we examine ATAC-Seq signal at Sp1 and brk loci in astrocyte-like glia ATAC-Seq, we find several peaks in both genes largely masked in heads, implying that they are subject to a unique mode of regulation in glia (Fig 7B). Thus, our data suggests the intriguing possibility that Sp1 and brk form a transcriptional pair specific to astrocyte-like glia and that many intrinsic cyclers in heads come from glia.

VibeCheck identifies common cycling genes across Clock neurons

A previous report from our group has found that the majority of rhythmic genes in subsets of Clock neurons are unique to each cluster, finding only about 350 genes that were shared between more than two clusters (Ma et al., 2021). We reexamined this claim using VibeCheck and a relatively high-stringency prediction value of 0.8 and found 769 transcripts shared between more than two clusters.

To find transcripts whose cycling is qualitatively shared between all clusters, we adjusted the thresholds for VibeCheck and manually examined plots for each gene that was classified as periodic or aperiodic following each adjustment. A threshold of 16 cell types and a prediction value of 0.4 revealed 47 genes that were qualitatively convincing in every cluster. These include validated core clock genes and CLK-direct target genes like *tim, vri, per, Pdp1, CG31324,* and *cwo* (Table 1). Interestingly, including the core clock genes, 11/47 are transcription factors – two such examples, HmgZ and chn, are shown in Fig 8A. These two genes are strikingly arrhythmic in heads (Fig 8B). In fact, of the 47 universal cyclers, only 10 of them are also cycling in heads. Aside from the core clock genes, the other common cyclers are *CG32369*, *CG44247*, *Cyt-c-p*, and *Eip63F-1*. *CG32369* is somewhat remarkable by merit of its loci being sandwich between *clk* and *Pdp1*; the rest have unknown circadian relationships.

Table 1: 47 genes cycling in every Clock neuron cell type

Act5C	CG1607	CG4577	Hipk	amon	nrv3
Ald1	CG31324	CG6329	HmgZ	bru3	pHCl-1
Argk	CG31808	CG6959	Pdp1	chinmo	per
Atpalpha	CG32264	CG9674	Pka-R1	chn	ringer
Bacc	CG32369	Clk	PyK	cwo	sesB
CG1090	CG32432	Cyt-c-p	Rbfox1	fne	tim
CG14082	CG43066	Dscam4	Sdc	jeb	vri
CG15628	CG44247	Eip63F-1	Unc-76	meng	

VibeCheck identifies unique cycling genes across Clock neuron clusters

While the number of common cycling genes is higher than originally reported, the observation that many cyclers are unique to individual clusters also holds true. We used an aggressive thresholding strategy to identify cluster-specific cyclers with high confidence. We defined background cyclers as genes with a Prediction Value of over 0.1 in at least 3 clusters, and unique cyclers as genes with a Prediction Value of over 0.75 in just 1 cluster. Using these conservative thresholds, we identified anywhere between 5 to 60 high confidence cluste r-specific cyclers (Fig 9A). The LNvs and the DN1p_1s have the most unique cyclers by far – over twice as many as any other cluster. This may be biological, but it also may be attributed to the fact that these two clusters also feature the most cells out of any other cluster, and that other clusters were not sequenced to saturating depths.

We sought to determine whether we could identify transcription factors potentially mediating cluster-specific cycling. First, we identified ATAC-Seq peaks in 856-GAL4 labeled cells – AKA Clock neurons - and subsetted peaks adjacent to uniquely cycling genes to identify gene-adjacent regulatory regions. We next performed a motif search across these regions using Homer and MEME to search for evidence of transcription factors regulating these genes.

We identified a distinct motif signature associated with uniquely cycling genes in four clusters. The first was identified in DN1p_1s and was a high confidence match to the Mad motif ($q < 0.05$) (Fig 9B). When examining Mad cycling across all clusters, DN1p_1s exhibited the clearest cycling with the highest amplitude. The second, identified in LPN_1s, was the Mitf motif ($q < 0.05$) (Fig 9C). Mitf exhibits some evidence of cycling in a handful of clusters, but the LPN_1s appear to have a relatively high amplitude. The third, identified in DN1p_7s was the bab1 motif ($q <0.05$) (Fig 9D). While bab1 appears to exhibit evidence of cycling in the DN1p_3s and DN1p_4s as well, it appears to exhibit a higher amplitude in the DN1p_7s. The fourth, identified in DN1as, is the klu motif – although the motif is not a perfect match to the known motif, and is not statistically significant following multiple hypothesis correction ($q > 0.05$) (Fig 9E). However, klu cycling indeed appears to be restricted to the DN1as – which encourages the possibility that klu is responsible for mediating rhythmic expression of DN1a-specific cyling genes. The klu motif was determined through Bacterial 1-hybrid experiments, and perhaps endogenous motif recognition may differ slightly.

These coincident observations suggests that these transcription factors may be responsible for conferring cell-type specific cycling in Clock neurons and merit further investigation.

DISCUSSION

In this study, we describe the development and employment of a novel neural network, VibeCheck, to identify rhythmicity from high-throughput transcriptomics data. VibeCheck is distinguished by its employment of an LSTM-based architecture with an attention layer in addition to a preprocessing circular encoding step. Together, these features render it highly adept at robustly identifying rhythmicity, even in high-noise data.

VibeCheck is optimized for identifying potential rhythmicity from data with a 4-hour sampling resolution – or in other words, sparsely sampled data. It represents a powerful tool for extracting hypotheses that may be concealed by existing approaches; however, as with any tool, it has significant limitations.

VibeCheck is not intended to return a definitive list of cycling genes. For such an exercise, there is no substitute for adequate sampling regimes. However, we demonstrate VibeCheck's potential for comparative circadian transcriptomics and identify several novel features of molecular rhythms, demonstrating it to be a powerful tool for hypothesis generation.

We show that by intersecting multiple "around-the-clock" datasets from *Drosophila* heads, we were able to identify a convincing list of cycling genes common to the majority of datasets – 511 in total. This represents a 2-fold improvement over the previous effort at identifying commonly cycling genes. The majority of these genes - 70% - further exhibited evidence of cycling at a transcriptional level, which corroborates a previous report (Atger et al., 2015). We leverage these common cyclers against ATAC-Seq data to identify a putative circadian network in astrocyte-like glia regulated by *Sp1* and *brk*.

We also demonstrate another potential use-case for VibeCheck by using it to explore differential rhythmicity in single-cell RNA-Seq from Clock neurons. By using a relaxed threshold for the reference set and a high threshold for the cell type of interest, we were able to identify many uniquely cycling genes with high confidence from each cell type. Four of these clusters were further distinguished by regulatory motifs implicating transcription factors potentially responsible for driving cell-type-specific cycling.

Throughout each exercise, regardless of what tool we used, we validated reports of cycling with plotting and manual examination. No approach was immune from false positives or false negatives, and every approach required us to tune our thresholds in order to produce a set of convincingly oscillating genes. Indeed, this and many other studies have found that reports of differential rhythmicity have been greatly exaggerated – something which might have been avoided had the investigators had simply plotted their data. We found this manual method unavoidable and invaluable. In other words, one might think of VibeCheck as a tool to reduce the number of genes one will have to plot and manually examine.

METHODS

RNA-Seq data processing.

RNA-Seq data used in this study are listed in supplementary table 1. Fastq files were retrieved from GEO using fasterq-dump. Reads from the same sample but multiple sequencing runs were merged prior to alignment. *Mus musculus* datasets used are listed in supplementary table 1. *Drosophila melanogaster* datasets used are listed in supplementary table 2.

A Salmon transcriptome index was constructed using the GRCm39 *Mus musculus* genome assembly using the entire genome as a decoy and the Gencode M32 transcriptome (Patro et al., 2017). Pseudoalignment and quantification was done using Salmon and standard parameters.

Counts were imported into R using the Tximeta package and transcript-level counts were summarized to gene-level counts, following best practices for RNA-seq quantification. Length and ratio of means normalized counts were obtained using DESeq2 (Love et al., 2014). Any gene where at least half the reads measured 0 were discarded.

Normalized counts were then normalized to 1 by dividing the counts for each gene by the highest value across all timepoints and replicates. Normalization was done across replicates and not within replicates to preserve the variation across replicates.

Cycling Analysis

JTK Cycle analysis was done using meta2d using default parameters (Wu et al., 2016). A p-value threshold of $BH.Q < 0.05$ was used to define cycling. No amplitude threshold was employed. RAIN analysis was conducted using peak.border set to 0.3 and 0.7 and a period of 24 (Thaben & Westermark, 2014). A p-value threshold of 0.05 was used to define rhythmicity.

Intersection simulation

Intersection simulation was conducted using a custom python script. Briefly, specificity and sensitivity parameters were set as previously reported. A set of true labels were set for simulated genes as oscillating or not oscillating, then a cycling analysis result was randomly generated according to the previously set sensitivity parameters. After simulating all experiments, we find genes that appear in at least X number of experiments and counts the number of true positives, false positives, and false negatives.

Training data for VibeCheck

Based on the results of intersection simulation, we defined a set of oscillating genes as genes that were cycling in at least 5 datasets for JTK Cycle and at least 14 datasets for RAIN. Genes in each individual dataset with a P-value < 0.05 not on the defined set of oscillating genes were removed from the training data. We reasoned that these may be environmentally influenced oscillating genes that may hinder VibeCheck's ability to generalize the training data.

VibeCheck data preprocessing

All transcriptomic datasets normalized to 1 were processed using a standardized pipeline for input into VibeCheck using Python. Each dataset was padded with -2 to make all datasets of even length – a value that is subsequently masked during training.

To emphasize the circular nature of circadian data, we used a circular encoding strategy. Each timepoint was transformed into two coordinates using sine and cosine functions, thus representing each measurement as a point on a unit circle with a 24-hour period.

Model Architecture

Our neural network model was constructed using TensorFlow 2.6.0 and Keras 2.6.0 libraries. An initial model consisting of a long short-term memory (LSTM) layer with 32 units and a tanh activation function, a dense layer with 32 units and a relu activation function, and a final dense layer with a single unit and a sigmoid activation function were used to tune the batch size and the learning rate. VibeCheck is compiled with an Adam optimizer and a binary cross-entropy loss function. An early stopping parameter with a patience of 8 was included as well.

Subsequent hyperparameter tuning was conducted for the number of layers, types of layers, number of units, activation functions, and dropout.

Throughout hyperparameter tuning, we tracked loss, accuracy, precision, recall, AUC, and F1 score.

Synthetic Data Generation

Synthetic data was generated using CircaInSilico using the following parameters: a maximum amplitude of 6, a minimum amplitude of 0.5, an outlier amplitude of 10, 4-hour resolution, 2 replicates, 15,000 genes, and 1,500 oscillating genes. Noise was adding using a custom Python script (Hughes et al., 2017).

ATAC-Seq Preprocessing

ATAC-Seq files were adaptor-trimmed using fastq. Bowtie2 was used to aligned trimmed files using the following parameters: --local --very-sensitive-local --no-unal --no-mixed --no-discordant --phred33 -I 10 -X 700 (Langmead & Salzberg, 2012). Samtools was used to remove PCR duplicates and Sambamba was used to remove multimapping reads (Li et al., 2009). Tn5 insertion bias was corrected using a custom python script and peaks were called using MACS2 (Zhang et al., 2008).

ATAC-Seq differential peak calling and normalization

Peaks called from MACS2 were intersected between replicates using bedtools, and peaks across conditions were merged and converted into a reference annotation in SAF format (Quinlan, 2014). Featurecounts was used to count reads in each sample within each region in the reference file, and input into DESeq2 in R. DESeq2 was used to perform differential peak quantification, and normalization factors were produced as well.

Normalization factors were used to produce normalize bigwig files for visualization using Deeptools bamcoverage (Ramirez et al., 2014).

Metagene plots were generated using Deeptools ComputeMatrix and PlotProfile.

ATAC-Seq Footprinting

Footprinting was conducted using TOBIAS (Bentsen et al., 2020). Briefly, footprints were retrieved from BAMfiles using ATACorrect and FootPrintScores. BINDetect was then used to compare footprinting between conditions. Motif databases from OnTheFly and JASPAR were used (Castro-Mondragon et al., 2022; Shazman et al., 2014).

Motif Analysis

ATAC-Seq peaks were annotated to their closest gene using bedtools. For HOMER, a bed file of peaks corresponding to genes of interest were directly input for motif analysis, with the original unfiltered peaks file being used as a background (Heinz et al., 2010). For MEME-ChIP, summit files from MACS2 were expanded 250nt in either direction using bedtools slop, and then fasta sequences corresponding to each coordinate was retrieved using bedtools getfasta. Fasta files were then submitted into MEME-ChIP for analysis (Bailey et al., 2015).

REFERENCES

Abruzzi, K. C., Rodriguez, J., Menet, J. S., Desrochers, J., Zadina, A., Luo, W., Tkachev, S., & Rosbash, M. (2011). Drosophila CLOCK target gene characterization: implications for circadian tissue-specific gene expression. *Genes Dev*, *25*(22), 2374-2386. https://doi.org/10.1101/gad.174110.111
10.1101/gad.178079.111

Agostinelli, F., Ceglia, N., Shahbaba, B., Sassone-Corsi, P., & Baldi, P. (2016). What time is it? Deep learning approaches for circadian rhythms. *Bioinformatics*, *32*(12), i8-i17. https://doi.org/10.1093/bioinformatics/btw243

Andreani, T. S., Itoh, T. Q., Yildirim, E., Hwangbo, D. S., & Allada, R. (2015). Genetics of Circadian Rhythms. *Sleep Med Clin*, *10*(4), 413-421. https://doi.org/10.1016/j.jsmc.2015.08.007

Atger, F., Gobet, C., Marquis, J., Martin, E., Wang, J., Weger, B., Lefebvre, G., Descombes, P., Naef, F., & Gachon, F. (2015). Circadian and feeding rhythms differentially affect rhythmic mRNA transcription and translation in mouse liver. *Proc Natl Acad Sci U S A*, *112*(47), E6579-6588. https://doi.org/10.1073/pnas.1515308112

Bailey, T. L., Johnson, J., Grant, C. E., & Noble, W. S. (2015). The MEME Suite. *Nucleic Acids Res*, *43*(W1), W39-49. https://doi.org/10.1093/nar/gkv416

Bentsen, M., Goymann, P., Schultheis, H., Klee, K., Petrova, A., Wiegandt, R., Fust, A., Preussner, J., Kuenne, C., Braun, T., Kim, J., & Looso, M. (2020). ATAC-seq footprinting unravels kinetics of transcription factor binding during zygotic genome activation. *Nat Commun*, *11*(1), 4267. https://doi.org/10.1038/s41467-020-18035-1

Heinz, S., Benner, C., Spann, N., Bertolino, E., Lin, Y. C., Laslo, P., Cheng, J. X., Murre, C., Singh, H., & Glass, C. K. (2010). Simple combinations of lineage-determining transcription factors prime cis-regulatory elements required for macrophage and B cell identities. *Mol Cell*, *38*(4), 576-589. https://doi.org/10.1016/j.molcel.2010.05.004

Hughes, M. E., Abruzzi, K. C., Allada, R., Anafi, R., Arpat, A. B., Asher, G., Baldi, P., de Bekker, C., Bell-Pedersen, D., Blau, J., Brown, S., Ceriani, M. F., Chen, Z., Chiu, J. C., Cox, J., Crowell, A. M., DeBruyne, J. P., Dijk, D. J., DiTacchio, L., . . . Hogenesch, J. B. (2017). Guidelines for Genome-Scale Analysis of Biological Rhythms. *J Biol Rhythms*, *32*(5), 380-393. https://doi.org/10.1177/0748730417728663

Hughes, M. E., DiTacchio, L., Hayes, K. R., Vollmers, C., Pulivarthy, S., Baggs, J. E., Panda, S., & Hogenesch, J. B. (2009). Harmonics of circadian gene transcription in mammals. *PLoS Genet*, *5*(4), e1000442. https://doi.org/10.1371/journal.pgen.1000442

Hughes, M. E., Hogenesch, J. B., & Kornacker, K. (2010). JTK_CYCLE: an efficient nonparametric algorithm for detecting rhythmic components in genome-scale data sets. *J Biol Rhythms*, *25*(5), 372-380. https://doi.org/10.1177/0748730410379711

Hutchison, A. L., Allada, R., & Dinner, A. R. (2018). Bootstrapping and Empirical Bayes Methods Improve Rhythm Detection in Sparsely Sampled Data. *J Biol Rhythms*, *33*(4), 339-349. https://doi.org/10.1177/0748730418789536

Keegan, K. P., Pradhan, S., Wang, J. P., & Allada, R. (2007). Meta-analysis of Drosophila circadian microarray studies identifies a novel set of rhythmically expressed genes. *PLoS Comput Biol*, *3*(11), e208. https://doi.org/10.1371/journal.pcbi.0030208

Koike, N., Yoo, S. H., Huang, H. C., Kumar, V., Lee, C., Kim, T. K., & Takahashi, J. S. (2012). Transcriptional architecture and chromatin landscape of the core circadian clock in mammals. *Science*, *338*(6105), 349-354. https://doi.org/10.1126/science.1226339

Li, H., Janssens, J., De Waegeneer, M., Kolluru, S. S., Davie, K., Gardeux, V., Saelens, W., David, F. P. A., Brbic, M., Spanier, K., Leskovec, J., McLaughlin, C. N., Xie, Q., Jones, R. C., Brueckner, K., Shim, J., Tattikota, S. G., Schnorrer, F., Rust, K., . . . Zinzen, R. P. (2022). Fly Cell Atlas: A single-nucleus transcriptomic atlas of the adult fruit fly. *Science*, *375*(6584), eabk2432. https://doi.org/10.1126/science.abk2432

Ma, D., Przybylski, D., Abruzzi, K. C., Schlichting, M., Li, Q., Long, X., & Rosbash, M. (2021). A transcriptomic taxonomy of Drosophila circadian neurons around the clock. *Elife*, *10*. https://doi.org/10.7554/eLife.63056

Mendez-Ferrer, S., Lucas, D., Battista, M., & Frenette, P. S. (2008). Haematopoietic stem cell release is regulated by circadian oscillations. *Nature*, *452*(7186), 442-447. https://doi.org/10.1038/nature06685

Ness-Cohn, E., Iwanaszko, M., Kath, W. L., Allada, R., & Braun, R. (2020). TimeTrial: An Interactive Application for Optimizing the Design and Analysis of Transcriptomic Time-Series Data in Circadian Biology Research. *J Biol Rhythms*, *35*(5), 439-451. https://doi.org/10.1177/0748730420934672

Patke, A., Young, M. W., & Axelrod, S. (2020). Molecular mechanisms and physiological importance of circadian rhythms. *Nat Rev Mol Cell Biol*, *21*(2), 67-84. https://doi.org/10.1038/s41580-019-0179-2

Pelikan, A., Herzel, H., Kramer, A., & Ananthasubramaniam, B. (2022). Venn diagram analysis overestimates the extent of circadian rhythm reprogramming. *FEBS J*, *289*(21), 6605-6621. https://doi.org/10.1111/febs.16095

Rodriguez, J., Tang, C. H., Khodor, Y. L., Vodala, S., Menet, J. S., & Rosbash, M. (2013). Nascent-Seq analysis of

Drosophila cycling gene expression. *Proc Natl Acad Sci U S A*, *110*(4), E275-284.
https://doi.org/10.1073/pnas.1219969110

Shokri, L., Inukai, S., Hafner, A., Weinand, K., Hens, K., Vedenko, A., Gisselbrecht, S. S., Dainese, R., Bischof, J., Furger, E., Feuz, J. D., Basler, K., Deplancke, B., & Bulyk, M. L. (2019). A Comprehensive Drosophila melanogaster Transcription Factor Interactome. *Cell Rep*, *27*(3), 955-970 e957.
https://doi.org/10.1016/j.celrep.2019.03.071

Thaben, P. F., & Westermark, P. O. (2014). Detecting rhythms in time series with RAIN. *J Biol Rhythms*, *29*(6), 391-400. https://doi.org/10.1177/0748730414553029

Wu, G., Anafi, R. C., Hughes, M. E., Kornacker, K., & Hogenesch, J. B. (2016). MetaCycle: an integrated R package to evaluate periodicity in large scale data. *Bioinformatics*, *32*(21), 3351-3353.
https://doi.org/10.1093/bioinformatics/btw405

Yu, A. D., & Rosbash, M. (2023). Butt-seq: a new method for facile profiling of transcription. *Genes Dev*, *37*(9-10), 432-448. https://doi.org/10.1101/gad.350434.123

FIGURES AND FIGURE LEGENDS

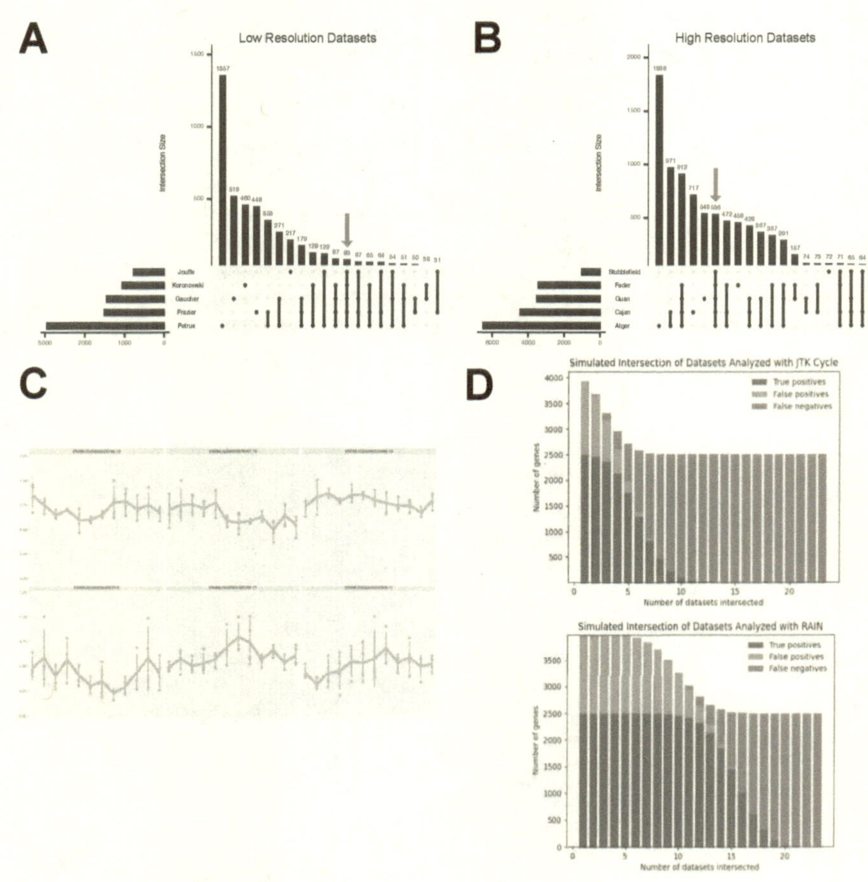

Figure 1. Examinations of cycling dynamics.

(A) Comparison of rhythmic transcripts in relatively sparsely sampled datasets. Datasets shown feature 4-hour sampling resolutions with 3 replicates. 2 replicate datasets with such sampling resolution typically had too few significantly cycling genes for meaningful comparison.

(B) Comparison of rhythmic transcripts in high sampling resolution datasets. Atger features 2 hour resolution with 4 replicates, Cajan has 2 hour resolution with 2 replicates, Guan and Fader have 3 hour resolution with 3 replicates, and Stubblefield has 2 hour resolution with 3 replicates.

(C) Significantly cycling (BH.Q < 0.05) transcripts from the Atger dataset with qualitatively absent cycling.

(D) Simulations of overlapping oscillating genes from JTK_Cycle (top) and RAIN (bottom) using sensitivity and specificity reported by Ness-Cohn et al., 2020.

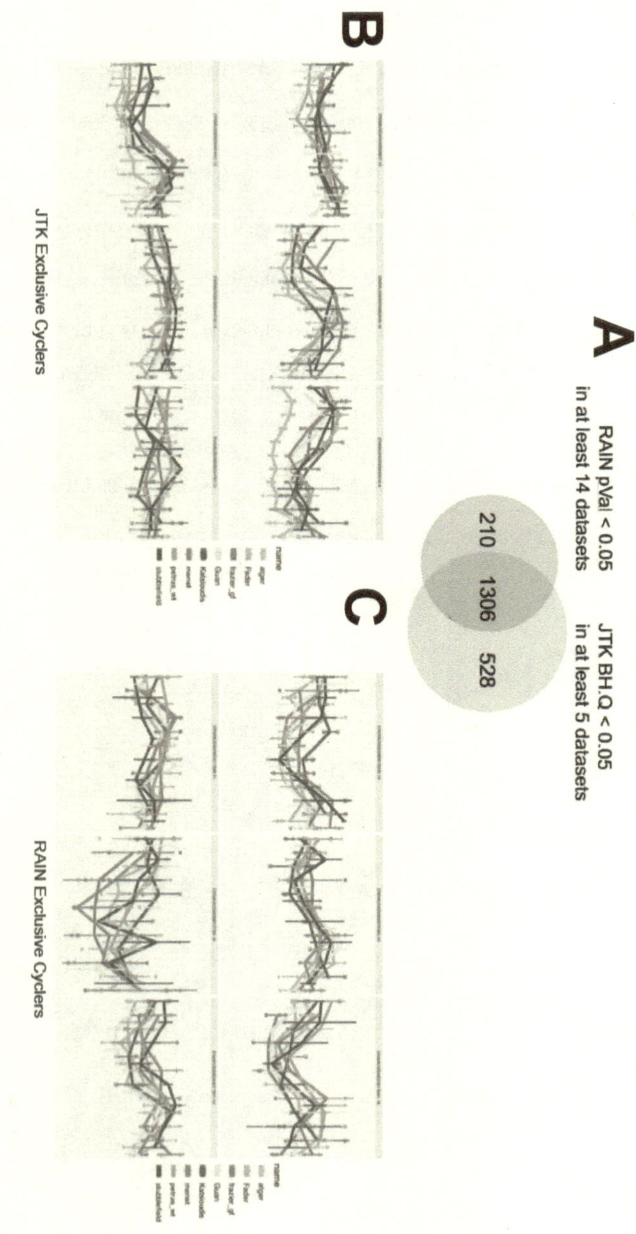
A
RAIN pVal < 0.05
in at least 14 datasets
210
1306
528
JTK BH.Q < 0.05
in at least 5 datasets
B
C
JTK Exclusive Cyclers
RAIN Exclusive Cyclers

Figure 2. Identifying common rhythmic genes between RAIN and JTK_Cycle

(A)Number of overlapping and unique genes between RAIN and JTK_Cycle.

(B)6 representative genes out of the 528 common cycling genes only called by JTK_Cycle. Only 8 out of 23 datasets are shown to maintain clarity.

(C)6 representative genes out of the 210 common cycling genes only called by RAIN. Only 8 out of 23 datasets are shown to maintain clarity.

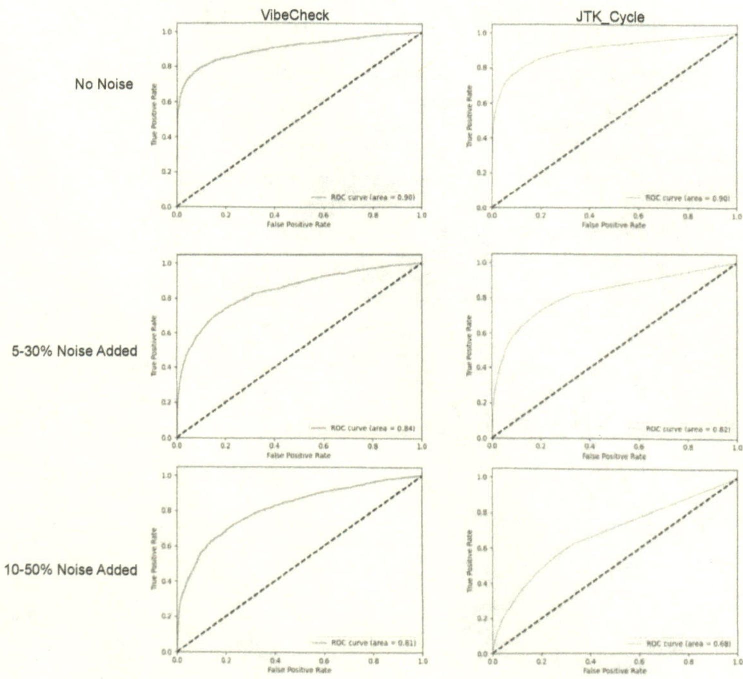

Figure 3. Benchmarking VibeCheck against JTK_Cycle on simulated data.

All 3 synthetic datasets were generated with CircalnSilico using a maximum amplitude of 6, a minimum amplitude of 0.5, an outlier amplitude of 10, 4-hour resolution, 2 replicates, 15,000 genes, and 1,500 oscillating genes.

Receiver operating characteristic (ROC) are plotted and area under curve (AUC) are reported for cycling analysis on standard CircalnSilico outputs (top), with 5-30% noise added (middle), and with 10-50% noise added (bottom).

A
VibeCheck Prediction > 0.5
in at least 5 datasets
JTK pValue < 0.05
in at least 5 datasets
380
132
1
Common Cyclers
Revealed by Vibecheck
B
name
Kuintzle_Young
Kuintzle_Old
Rivas
Rodriguez
SebTG4
Wang_Young
C
name
Kuintzle_Young
Rivas
Rodriguez
SebTG4
Wang_Young

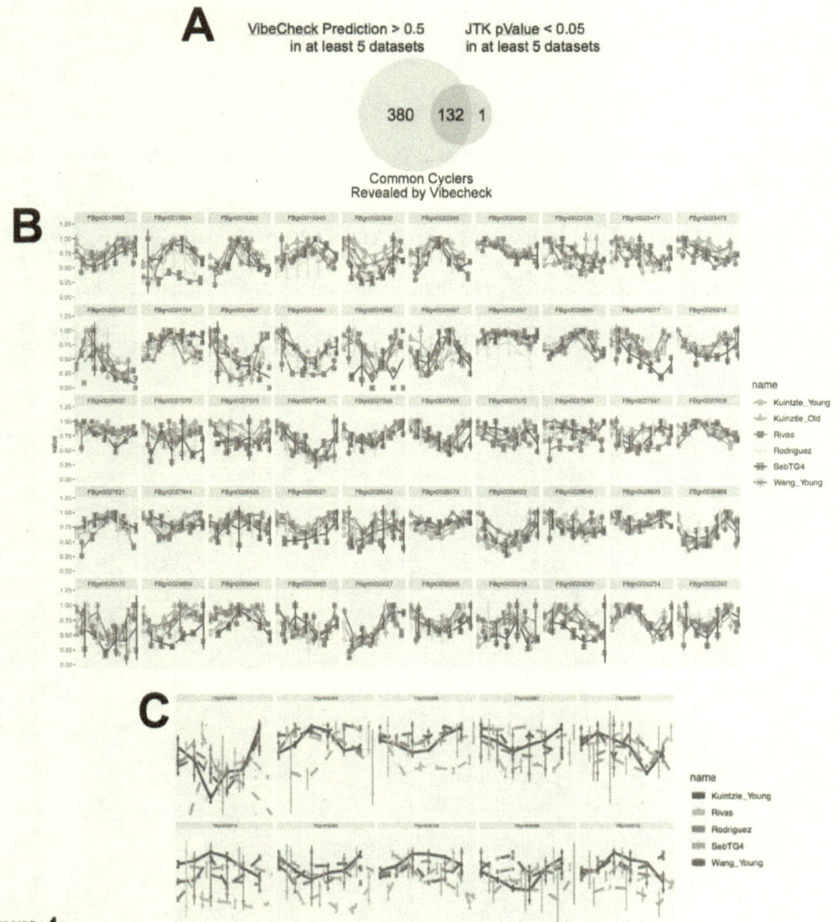

Figure 4

Figure 4. Analysis of circadian dynamics in *D. Melanogaster* heads using VibeCheck and JTK_Cycle.

(A) Venn diagram of oscillating transcripts as determined by VibeCheck and JTK_Cycle.

(B) 50 representative genes called as oscillating transcripts determined by VibeCheck

(C) 10 representative genes that were only reported as cycling Kuintzle dataset by both VibeCheck and JTK_Cycle

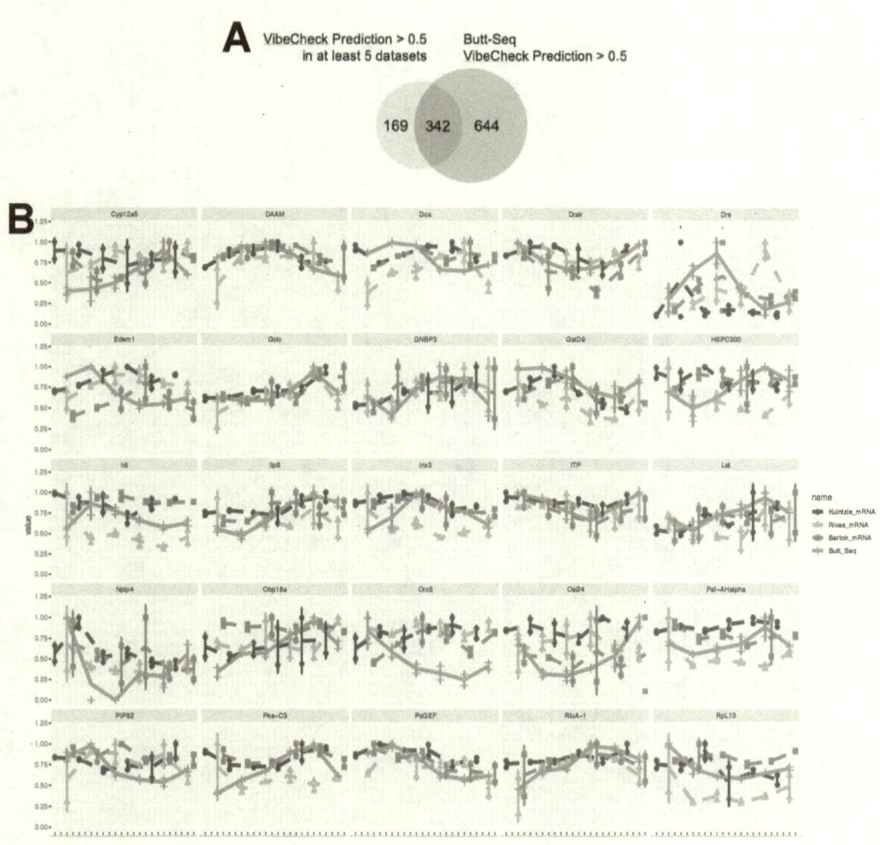

Figure 5. Comparison of oscillations between mRNA and nascent RNA as measured by Butt-Seq.

(A) Overlap of oscillating transcripts between mRNA and Butt-Seq as determined by VibeCheck

(B) 25 representative genes oscillating in Butt-Seq not previously found to be reproducibly cycling in mRNA-seq data.

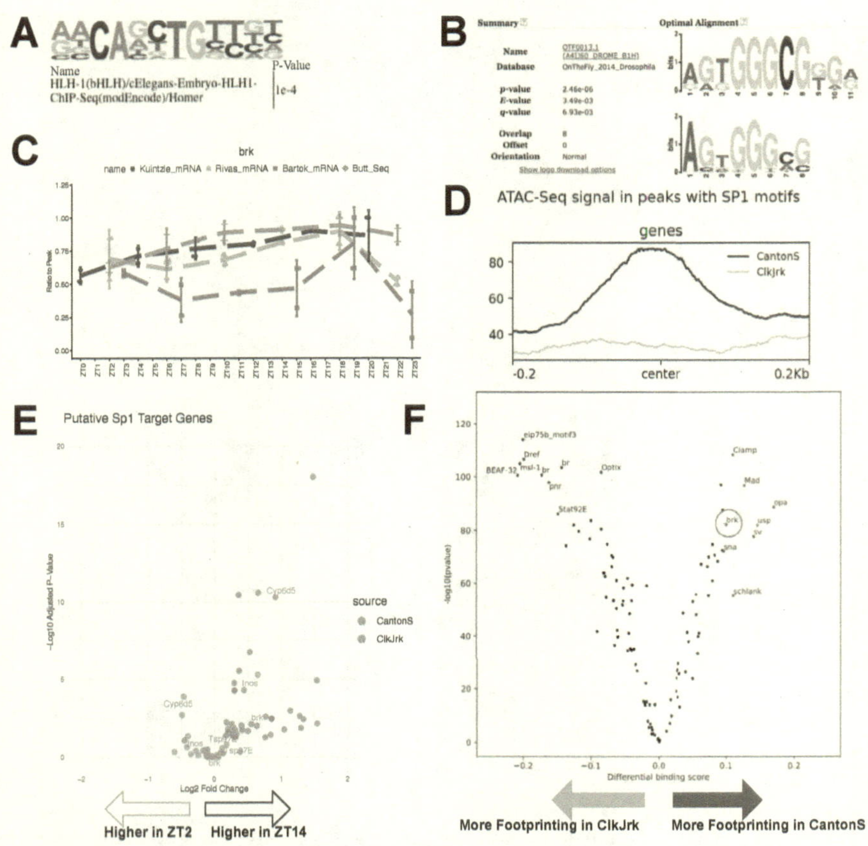
A
Name
HLH-1(bHLH)/cElegans-Embryo-HLH1-ChIP-Seq(modEncode)/Homer
P-Value
1e-4
B
Summary
Optimal Alignment
Name
Database
OnTheFly_2014_Drosophila
p-value
E-value
q-value
Overlap
Offset
Orientation
Normal
C
brk
name Kuintzle_mRNA Rivas_mRNA Bartok_mRNA Butt_Seq
Ratio to Peak
D
ATAC-Seq signal in peaks with SP1 motifs
genes
CantonS
Clkjrk
-0.2
center
0.2Kb
E
Putative Sp1 Target Genes
-Log10 Adjusted P-Value
Log2 Fold Change
source
CantonS
ClkJrk
Cyp6d5
Inos
brk
Higher in ZT2
Higher in ZT14
F
eip75b_motif3
Dref
BEAF-32
msl-1
br
pnr
Optix
Stat92E
Clamp
Mad
opa
brk
usp
sv
sna
schlank
-log10(pvalue)
Differential binding score
More Footprinting in ClkJrk
More Footprinting in CantonS

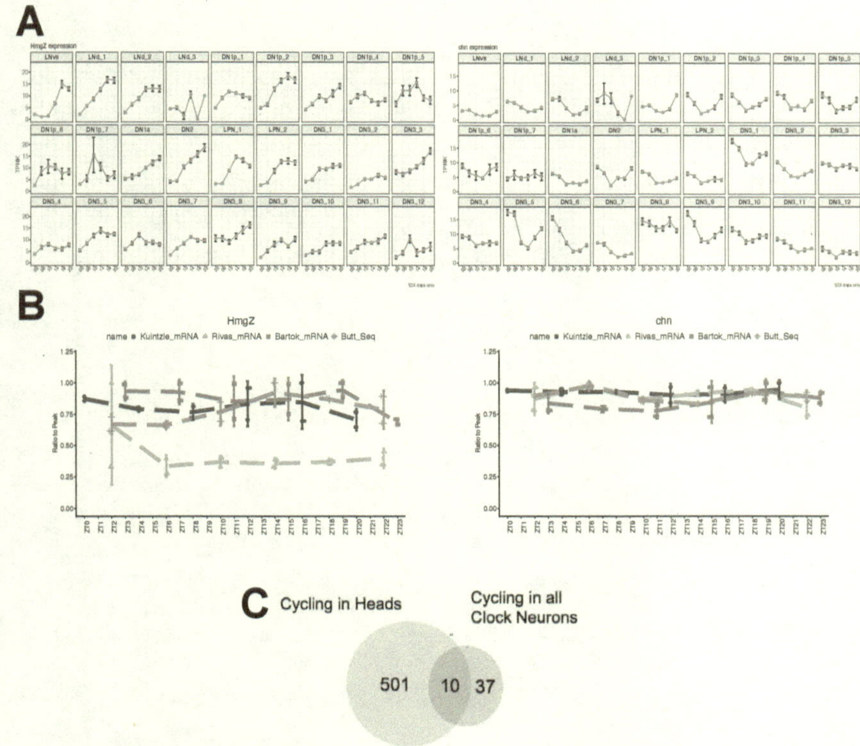

Figure 8. Identification of common cycling genes between different cell types among Clock neurons.

(A) 2 transcription factors plotted across 6 timepoints in 27 cell types from single-cell RNA sequencing data from Clock neurons. HmgZ (left) and chn (right).

(B) The same transcription factors from (A) plotted from head mRNA-Seq (green, purple, and blue) and Butt-Seq (pink). HmgZ (left) and chn (right).

(C) Venn diagram of commonly cycling genes in heads and clock neurons.

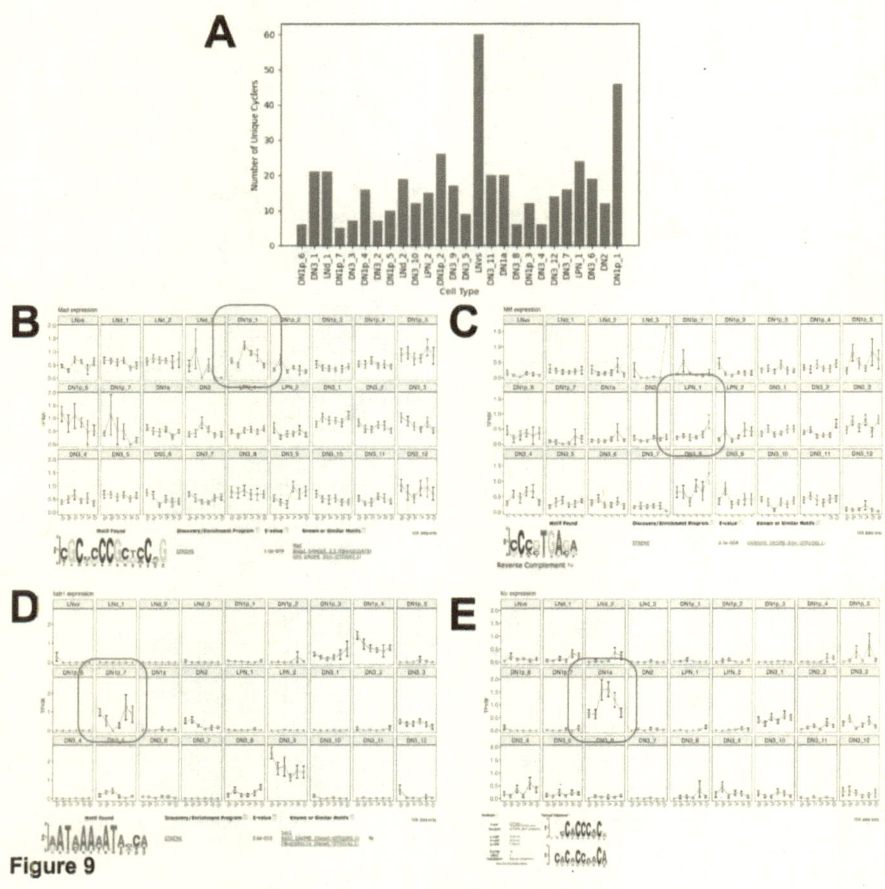

A
Number of Unique Cyclers
0
10
20
30
40
50
60
DN1p_6
DN3_1
LNd_1
DN1p_7
DN3_3
DN1p_4
DN3_2
DN1p_5
LNd_2
DN3_10
LPN_2
DN1p_2
DN3_9
DN3_5
LNvs
DN3_11
DN1a
DN3_8
DN1p_3
DN3_4
DN3_12
DN3_7
LPN_1
DN3_6
DN2
DN1p_1
Cell Type
B
C
D
E

Figure 9

Figure 9. Features of cell-type specific cycling genes in Clock neurons.

(A) Number of uniquely cycling genes in each clock neuron.

(B) The *mad* motif identified in regulatory regions in genes only cycling DN1p_1s (bottom). Expression of *mad* across 27 cell types in Clock neurons from single-cell RNA-sequencing (top). DN1p_1s are circled in pink.

(C) The *Mitf* motif identified in regulatory regions in genes only cycling LPN_1s (bottom). Expression of *Mitf* across 27 cell types in Clock neurons from single-cell RNA-sequencing (top). LPN_1s are circled in pink.

(D) The *bab1* motif identified in regulatory regions in genes only cycling DN1p_7s (bottom). Expression of *bab1* across 27 cell types in Clock neurons from single-cell RNA-sequencing (top). DN1p_7s are circled in pink.

(E) The *klu* motif identified in regulatory regions in genes only cycling DN1as (bottom). Expression of *klu* across 27 cell types in Clock neurons from single-cell RNA-sequencing (top). DN1as are circled in pink.

Name	Corresponding Author	GEO ID	Sampling Resolution (Hours)	# of replicates
Cajan	Naef	GSE61775	2	2
Atger	Gachon	GSE73554	2	4
Guan	Lazar	GSE143528	3	3
Fader	Zacharewski	GSE119780	3	3
Stubblefield	Green	GSE105413	3	2
Mezhnina_AL	Kondratov	GSE211975	4	3
Petrus_WT	Benitah	GSE196430	4	3
Katsioudis	Gatfield	GSE208769	4	3
Astafev_AL	Kondratov	GSE216416	4	3
Frazier	Chang	GSE184303	4	3
Weger	Naef	GSE135898	4	2
Gaucher	Sassone-Corsi	GSE132103	4	3
Abe	Fukada	GSE199061	4	2
Koronowski2019	Sassone-Corsi	GSE117134	4	3
Koronowski	Sassone-Corsi	GSE158600	4	3
Jouffe	Gachon	GSE190221	4	2
Greenwell	Menet	GSE118967	4	3
WegerBD	Gachon	GSE114400	4	2
Paschos	FitzGerald	GSE70499	4	3
Yang	Chen	GSE70497	4	4
Menet	Rosbash	GSE36871	4	2
Greco	Sassone-Corsi	GSE171432	4	3

Supplementary Table 1: *Mus musculus* datasets used in this study.

imagined that everyone would be rushing to investigate whether their favorite transcription factor mediated pause release or initiation (Adelman & Lis, 2012).

Dozens of excellent studies have dissected mechanisms that promote or release pausing. However, the components outlined by these studies are almost exclusively RNAPII CTD interacting proteins; only a handful of studies implicate transcription factors with any gene specificity playing a role in pause release (Adelman et al., 2009; Galbraith et al., 2013; Gupte et al., 2013). This absence might be due to lack of interest – or it could indicate that the role of polymerase pausing was something more subtle (or both).

My contemplations on the role of polymerase pausing began to intersect with another interest of mine – chromatin topology. Chromatin topology has been a field of interest for decades, but I would argue that it truly came into vogue with the introduction of high-throughput sequencing. As an exciting new trend, I felt compelled to stay on top of the literature. As I consumed more polymerase pausing literature and chromatin topology literature, I started to cultivate a hypothesis that chromatin topology and polymerase pausing might be closely interlinked.

Chromatin topology subtly mediates gene expression and has a seemingly overlooked relationship with polymerase pausing

Topologically associated domains (TADs) are a feature of chromatin organization defined by distal regions of chromatin looping around and physically contacting one another (Beagan & Phillips-Cremins, 2020). Within the larger TAD are smaller, stably interacting domains which include enhancer-promoter and promoter-promoter contacts. The implications were full of possibility – distal regulatory regions could share transcription factors with one another, thereby establishing physical proximity as a mode of gene regulation invisible in the genetic code. Chromatin loops were hypothesized to be pivotal nexuses of gene regulation, coordinating gene expression on a massive scale (Dixon et al., 2012; Dowen et al., 2014). However, the truth turned out to be somewhat subtle – deletions and inversions of TAD boundaries only have a modest effect on gene expression (Despang et al., 2019). The current leading hypothesis seems to be that TADs exist to fine-tune coordinated gene expression. (I'd like to casually mention here that circadian rhythms are a fine example of coordinated gene expression.)

The first hints of 3D genome organization emerged in *D. melanogaster*, where the discovery of position-effect variegation hinted that genomic positioning played an important role in gene expression (Muller, 1930). Since then, many components mediating chromatin topology have been identified. They were mostly first identified as insulator proteins that demarcated genetic borders of gene regulation. Recently, some of these insulator proteins have been validated as mediators of chromatin topology, thanks to chromosome conformation capture technology (Schwartz & Cavalli, 2017). These include BEAF-32, M1BP/CP190, and GAF (encoded by the *trl* gene) – all within the past 4 years (Bag et al., 2021; Herman et al., 2022; Li et al., 2023).

In seems almost conspiratorial that, prior to their characterization as topology factors, these genes were first described to have a role in promoter-proximal pausing. The discovery of GAF's involvement in pausing occurred just a few years after the discovery of pausing itself (Lee et al., 1992). Later, M1BP's role in pausing would be described as well – one distinct from GAF (Li & Gilmour, 2013). Not only did they bind at distinct sites, but the dwell time of RNAPII was distinct between GAF-mediated and M1BP-mediated pause sites. Soon after that, another study noticed that pauses that were insensitive to GAF depletion were marked by either M1BP or BEAF-32 binding (Fuda et al., 2015).

At this point, it seems unimaginable that groups studying promoter-proximal pausing would not have made the connection between the dual roles of GAF, M1BP, and BEAF-32 in promoter-proximal pausing and chromatin topology – however, I can think of a few reasons why we haven't seen any studies linking the two phenomena yet.

First, these studies are very new – M1BP's role in topology was the first to be identified, and it was just published in 2021. Perhaps we are only a year or two away from someone doing a chromosome conformation experiment following inducible pause factor degradation *(Note: This has been published the day after I wrote this).*

Second: the study of chromatin topology factors in promoter-proximal pausing is almost completely exclusive to *D. melanogaster*, so it may suffer a lack of awareness outside of fruitfly labs.

Third, there aren't enough chromatin topology people in *D. melanogaster.* The number of studies investigating chromatin topology in *D. melanogaster* absolutely pales in comparison to the number of studies investigating mammalian topology. This seems like a particular injustice when considering that the very concept of chromatin topology was pioneered in *D. melanogaster*, not to mention *D. melanogaster's* smaller genome means substantially reduced experimental costs.

These points might lead you to believe evidence of polymerase pausing being linked to chromatin topology is exclusive to *D. melanogaster* – but there is some evidence this connection exists in mammals as well. Though the literature linking chromatin topology factors to polymerase pausing is weak (though not non-existent) in mammals, there have been at least two studies that implicate RNA as a chromatin tether (Shukla et al., 2011).

RNA is involved in enhancer-promoter contacts within TADs

M1BP, GAF, and BEAF-32 are required for both promoter-proximal pausing and chromatin loops – but are these functions independent of one another? I would hypothesize that they are not, and that maintenance of chromatin contacts are dependent on the RNA molecule emerging from the stalled polymerase. Two pieces of evidence implicating RNA as chromatin tether have emerged from mammalian studies.

In 2017, one such study describes the involvement of the transcription factor Yin Yang 1 (YY1) in mediating enhancer-promoter contacts (Weintraub et al., 2017). They report that YY1 is located at these contacts, that YY1 dimerizes, that YY1 binds both DNA and RNA, and that RNAse A treatment reduces YY1 occupancy on DNA. Thus, they describe a model where YY1 monomers bind both DNA and RNA on enhancers and promoters, then bring them together through dimerization.

3 years later, in 2020, another study broaches this possibility with a sledgehammer. They develop a technique called RNA in situ conformation sequencing (RIC-seq), which ligates together proximal RNA molecules, then sequences these chimeric RNA molecules to see what distal RNA molecules are in proximity with one another (Cai et al., 2020). They observed hundreds of contacts between nascent RNAs and enhancer RNAs and suggest that RNA may be involved in forming contacts between enhancers and promoters.

Much to my frustration, RIC-seq libraries are prepared with standard RNA-seq protocols with random hexamer reverse transcription and Gubler and Hoffman second-strand synthesis, the former limiting resolution from the 3' end of the RNA molecule and the latter limiting resolution at the 5' end (Gubler & Hoffman, 1983). These two steps will drop out almost all short RNA molecules generated by promoter-proximal pausing – even if they were chimeric. Had they instead used a small RNA library preparation method, I hypothesize that they would observe countless RNA-RNA contacts corresponding to promoter-proximal pausing.

Stable enhancer-promoter contacts are only found in organisms with promoter-proximal pausing

"Nothing in Biology Makes Sense Except in the Light of Evolution" – so says Theodosius Dobzhansky, and so does it apply here as well. There is evidence that promoter-proximal pausing and enhancer-promoter looping emerged through evolution hand-in-hand.

I first noticed myself that promoter-proximal pausing in Saccharomyces Cerevisiae appeared distinct from promoter-proximal pausing in D. melanogaster. NET-seq data from S. cerevisiae lacked the distinct, sharp pausing peak that I observed in Butt-Seq data, and instead, appeared smaller and more disperse. I first attributed this to differences in the two techniques – but a recent manuscript claims that promoter-proximal pausing is entirely absent in S. cerevisiae (Alexandra et al., 2023).

This study would go on to describe the presence or absence of pausing across many evolutionary lineages – noting that it's ubiquitous in metazoans, but completely absent from Arabidopsis Thaliana and S. cerevisiae and mostly absent in Saccharomyces pombe. They report that the presence of pausing is associated with the presence of negative elongation factor (NELF) genes – which, as the name suggests, negatively regulate pause release.

As it so happens, A. thaliana and S. cerevisiae also do not exhibit sub-TAD contacts in the same way metazoans do (Dong et al., 2020; Duan et al., 2010). These species appear to lack stable short-range promoter-promoter and enhancer-promoter contacts.

There is one remarkable and perhaps highly telling exception: Zea mays does not contain any NELF proteins but does exhibit promoter-proximal pausing and similar chromatin topology to NELF-bearing metazoans (Alexandra et al., 2023; Dong et al., 2020). For a species to evolve independent mechanisms of both polymerase pausing and enhancer-promoter contacts strikes me as unlikely – the parsimonious explanation is that the two are mechanistically connected.

Pause release depletes enhancer-promoter contacts

The evidence for a link between chromatin looping and polymerase pausing appears enormous, and I thought I couldn't have been the only one to notice. It turns out I had good reason to think so – a study was published at time of writing that describes precisely what I am hypothesizing. This study found that by transiently depleting NELF and releasing paused polymerase, they induced the loss of enhancer-promoter contacts genome-wide (Barshad et al., 2023). Restoring NELF expression rescued enhancer-promoter contacts, and thus demonstrated the dependency of enhancer-promoter contacts on polymerase pausing. This study was conducted with human cells, where, as I mentioned earlier, there is a dearth of evidence connecting topology factors to promoter-proximal pausing. I would bet that this mechanism is conserved in *D. melanogaster* as well.

Nevertheless, there are still many outstanding questions left to be answered – namely, what sort of biological mechanisms could be driven by this mode of regulation?

Circadian involvement of polymerase pausing and enhancer-promoter looping is an open question

A handful of studies have been performed examining the impact of chromatin topology on circadian rhythms (Aguilar-Arnal et al., 2013; Kim et al., 2018; Mermet et al., 2018; Yeung et al., 2018). Not surprisingly, these studies have mostly been limited in scope – the cost and difficulty of chromosome conformation experiments are high enough for one condition, much less 6 to 12. The largest study used two timepoints – ZT10 and ZT22 – and showed that repressive core clock gene Rev-erbα repressed enhancer-promoter contacts at ZT10.

Thus, I find that the role of chromatin topology in circadian rhythms to be a wide-open question. I have two pieces of evidence that suggest that chromatin topology and polymerase pausing play a role in circadian rhythms in *Drosophila*.

First, at least two investigators in the Rosbash lab have independently noted that circadian genes are marked by an abundance of GAF/*trl* motifs (one of them is me). The idea that they play a role in circadian transcription is a very tempting one.

Second, I direct you to Figure 6F in Chapter 4, where I examine transcription factor footprints from ATAC-seq data between CantonS and a ClkJrk (a clock mutant with no circadian rhythms). You'll notice that the *Clamp* motif (identical to the GAF/*trl* motif), is also reduced in ClkJrk, while BEAF-32 is increased. As I discussed earlier, both BEAF-32 and GAF are involved in chromatin topology and polymerase pausing, but they never co-localize. I expect this may be reflected in pausing through Butt-Seq – so expanding my search for changes in pausing informed by *trl* and *Beaf-32* motifs may be the first thing I do upon defending my thesis. Preliminary analysis suggests that this may prove a fruitful source of experimentally tractable polymerase pausing – not only promoter-proximal, but intronic as well.

Thus, to loop back to the beginning of the discussion, I would say that where I went wrong is that instead of trying to identify rhythmic pause release, perhaps I should instead look for evidence of adjacent oscillating genes around highly paused transcripts. This isn't an entirely new idea – the first microarray study to examine oscillating transcription in *D. melanogaster* noted that some oscillating transcripts were adjacent to one another (McDonald & Rosbash, 2001). Anyone who has stared at their circadian datasets on IGV has surely noticed that the region surrounding *Clk* are rife with oscillating transcripts. Preliminary analysis suggests that there are indeed patterns that can be identified from oscillating gene expression alone. Perhaps, then, pausing and chromatin looping work together to regulate coordinated transcription.

REFERENCES

Adelman, K., Kennedy, M. A., Nechaev, S., Gilchrist, D. A., Muse, G. W., Chinenov, Y., & Rogatsky, I. (2009). Immediate mediators of the inflammatory response are poised for gene activation through RNA polymerase II stalling. *Proc Natl Acad Sci U S A*, *106*(43), 18207-18212. https://doi.org/10.1073/pnas.0910177106

Adelman, K., & Lis, J. T. (2012). Promoter-proximal pausing of RNA polymerase II: emerging roles in metazoans. *Nat Rev Genet*, *13*(10), 720-731. https://doi.org/10.1038/nrg3293

Aguilar-Arnal, L., Hakim, O., Patel, V. R., Baldi, P., Hager, G. L., & Sassone-Corsi, P. (2013). Cycles in spatial and temporal chromosomal organization driven by the circadian clock. *Nat Struct Mol Biol*, *20*(10), 1206-1213. https://doi.org/10.1038/nsmb.2667

Alexandra, G. C., Abderhman, A., Gilad, B., Edward, J. R., Michelle, M. L., Albert, C. V., Wilfred, W., Rebecca, B., Jeramiah, J. S., Athula, H. W., César, A.-M., Ilana, L. B., Iñaki, R.-T., Anna-Katerina, H., John, T. L., James, J. L., & Charles, G. D. (2023). Evolution of promoter-proximal pausing enabled a new layer of transcription control. *bioRxiv*, 2023.2002.2019.529146. https://doi.org/10.1101/2023.02.19.529146

Bag, I., Chen, S., Rosin, L. F., Chen, Y., Liu, C. Y., Yu, G. Y., & Lei, E. P. (2021). M1BP cooperates with CP190 to activate transcription at TAD borders and promote chromatin insulator activity. *Nat Commun*, *12*(1), 4170. https://doi.org/10.1038/s41467-021-24407-y

Barshad, G., Lewis, J. J., Chivu, A. G., Abuhashem, A., Krietenstein, N., Rice, E. J., Ma, Y., Wang, Z., Rando, O. J., Hadjantonakis, A. K., & Danko, C. G. (2023). RNA polymerase II dynamics shape enhancer-promoter interactions. *Nat Genet*. https://doi.org/10.1038/s41588-023-01442-7

Beagan, J. A., & Phillips-Cremins, J. E. (2020). On the existence and functionality of topologically associating domains. *Nat Genet*, *52*(1), 8-16. https://doi.org/10.1038/s41588-019-0561-1

Cai, Z., Cao, C., Ji, L., Ye, R., Wang, D., Xia, C., Wang, S., Du, Z., Hu, N., Yu, X., Chen, J., Wang, L., Yang, X., He, S., & Xue, Y. (2020). RIC-seq for global in situ profiling of RNA-RNA spatial interactions. *Nature*, *582*(7812), 432-437. https://doi.org/10.1038/s41586-020-2249-1

Despang, A., Schopflin, R., Franke, M., Ali, S., Jerkovic, I., Paliou, C., Chan, W. L., Timmermann, B., Wittler, L., Vingron, M., Mundlos, S., & Ibrahim, D. M. (2019). Functional dissection of the Sox9-Kcnj2 locus identifies nonessential and instructive roles of TAD architecture. *Nat Genet*, *51*(8), 1263-1271. https://doi.org/10.1038/s41588-019-0466-z

Dixon, J. R., Selvaraj, S., Yue, F., Kim, A., Li, Y., Shen, Y., Hu, M., Liu, J. S., & Ren, B. (2012). Topological domains in mammalian genomes identified by analysis of chromatin interactions. *Nature*, *485*(7398), 376-380. https://doi.org/10.1038/nature11082

Dong, P., Tu, X., Liang, Z., Kang, B. H., & Zhong, S. (2020). Plant and animal chromatin three-dimensional organization: similar structures but different functions. *J Exp Bot*, *71*(17), 5119-5128. https://doi.org/10.1093/jxb/eraa220

Dowen, J. M., Fan, Z. P., Hnisz, D., Ren, G., Abraham, B. J., Zhang, L. N., Weintraub, A. S., Schujiers, J., Lee, T. I., Zhao, K., & Young, R. A. (2014). Control of cell identity genes occurs in insulated neighborhoods in mammalian chromosomes. *Cell*, *159*(2), 374-387. https://doi.org/10.1016/j.cell.2014.09.030

Duan, Z., Andronescu, M., Schutz, K., McIlwain, S., Kim, Y. J., Lee, C., Shendure, J., Fields, S., Blau, C. A., & Noble, W. S. (2010). A three-dimensional model of the yeast genome. *Nature*, *465*(7296), 363-367. https://doi.org/10.1038/nature08973

Fuda, N. J., Guertin, M. J., Sharma, S., Danko, C. G., Martins, A. L., Siepel, A., & Lis, J. T. (2015). GAGA factor maintains nucleosome-free regions and has a role in RNA polymerase II recruitment to promoters. *PLoS Genet*, *11*(3), e1005108. https://doi.org/10.1371/journal.pgen.1005108

Galbraith, M. D., Allen, M. A., Bensard, C. L., Wang, X., Schwinn, M. K., Qin, B., Long, H. W., Daniels, D. L., Hahn, W. C., Dowell, R. D., & Espinosa, J. M. (2013). HIF1A employs CDK8-mediator to stimulate RNAPII elongation in response to hypoxia. *Cell*, *153*(6), 1327-1339. https://doi.org/10.1016/j.cell.2013.04.048

Gubler, U., & Hoffman, B. J. (1983). A simple and very efficient method for generating cDNA libraries. *Gene*, *25*(2-3), 263-269. https://doi.org/10.1016/0378-1119(83)90230-5

Gupte, R., Muse, G. W., Chinenov, Y., Adelman, K., & Rogatsky, I. (2013). Glucocorticoid receptor represses proinflammatory genes at distinct steps of the transcription cycle. *Proc Natl Acad Sci U S A*, *110*(36), 14616-14621. https://doi.org/10.1073/pnas.1309898110

Herman, N., Kadener, S., & Shifman, S. (2022). The chromatin factor ROW cooperates with BEAF-32 in regulating long-range inducible genes. *EMBO Rep*, *23*(12), e54720. https://doi.org/10.15252/embr.202254720

Kim, Y. H., Marhon, S. A., Zhang, Y., Steger, D. J., Won, K. J., & Lazar, M. A. (2018). Rev-erbalpha dynamically

modulates chromatin looping to control circadian gene transcription. *Science*, *359*(6381), 1274-1277. https://doi.org/10.1126/science.aao6891
Lee, H., Kraus, K. W., Wolfner, M. F., & Lis, J. T. (1992). DNA sequence requirements for generating paused polymerase at the start of hsp70. *Genes Dev*, *6*(2), 284-295. https://doi.org/10.1101/gad.6.2.284
Li, J., & Gilmour, D. S. (2013). Distinct mechanisms of transcriptional pausing orchestrated by GAGA factor and M1BP, a novel transcription factor. *EMBO J*, *32*(13), 1829-1841. https://doi.org/10.1038/emboj.2013.111
Li, X., Tang, X., Bing, X., Catalano, C., Li, T., Dolsten, G., Wu, C., & Levine, M. (2023). GAGA-associated factor fosters loop formation in the Drosophila genome. *Mol Cell*, *83*(9), 1519-1526 e1514. https://doi.org/10.1016/j.molcel.2023.03.011
McDonald, M. J., & Rosbash, M. (2001). Microarray analysis and organization of circadian gene expression in Drosophila. *Cell*, *107*(5), 567-578. https://doi.org/10.1016/s0092-8674(01)00545-1
Mermet, J., Yeung, J., Hurni, C., Mauvoisin, D., Gustafson, K., Jouffe, C., Nicolas, D., Emmenegger, Y., Gobet, C., Franken, P., Gachon, F., & Naef, F. (2018). Clock-dependent chromatin topology modulates circadian transcription and behavior. *Genes Dev*, *32*(5-6), 347-358. https://doi.org/10.1101/gad.312397.118
Muller, H. J. (1930). Types of visible variations induced by X-rays inDrosophila. *Journal of Genetics*, *22*(3), 299-334. https://doi.org/10.1007/BF02984195
Schwartz, Y. B., & Cavalli, G. (2017). Three-Dimensional Genome Organization and Function in Drosophila. *Genetics*, *205*(1), 5-24. https://doi.org/10.1534/genetics.115.185132
Shukla, S., Kavak, E., Gregory, M., Imashimizu, M., Shutinoski, B., Kashlev, M., Oberdoerffer, P., Sandberg, R., & Oberdoerffer, S. (2011). CTCF-promoted RNA polymerase II pausing links DNA methylation to splicing. *Nature*, *479*(7371), 74-79. https://doi.org/10.1038/nature10442
Weintraub, A. S., Li, C. H., Zamudio, A. V., Sigova, A. A., Hannett, N. M., Day, D. S., Abraham, B. J., Cohen, M. A., Nabet, B., Buckley, D. L., Guo, Y. E., Hnisz, D., Jaenisch, R., Bradner, J. E., Gray, N. S., & Young, R. A. (2017). YY1 Is a Structural Regulator of Enhancer-Promoter Loops. *Cell*, *171*(7), 1573-1588 e1528. https://doi.org/10.1016/j.cell.2017.11.008
Yeung, J., Mermet, J., Jouffe, C., Marquis, J., Charpagne, A., Gachon, F., & Naef, F. (2018). Transcription factor activity rhythms and tissue-specific chromatin interactions explain circadian gene expression across organs. *Genome Res*, *28*(2), 182-191. https://doi.org/10.1101/gr.222430.117

www.ingramcontent.com/pod-product-compliance
Lightning Source LLC
LaVergne TN
LVHW090932150826
845672LV00006B/1485

* 9 7 8 3 3 8 4 2 5 9 6 1 5 *